At Home with Terminal Illness

A Family Guide to Hospice in the Home

MICHAEL APPLETON, M.D.
TODD HENSCHELL

Prentice Hall Career & Technology
Englewood Cliffs, New Jersey 07632

Library of Congress Cataloging in Publication Data

Appleton, Michael, (date)
  At home with terminal illness: a family guide to hospice in the
  home/Michael Appleton, Todd Henschell.
     p.   cm.
  ISBN 0-13-299843-2
  1. Terminally ill—home care. 2. Hospice care. I. Henschell,
Todd. II. Title.
R726.8.A66   1995
362.1'75—dc20   94–9604

Acquisitions Editor: MARK HARTMAN
Editorial Assistant: LOUISE FULLAM
Director of Production Services: DAVID RICCARDI
Production Coordinator: ILENE LEVY SANFORD
Page Layout: JEFFERSON HARMAN
Cover Art: MERLE KRUMPER
Cover Design: WENDY HELFT, DESIGN W

© 1995 by Prentice Hall Career & Technology
Prentice-Hall, Inc.
A Paramount Communications Company
Englewood Cliffs, New Jersey 07632

Printed in the United States of America
1 2 3 4 5 6 7 8 9 10

ISBN: 0-13-299843-2

Prentice-Hall International (UK) Limited, *London*
Prentice-Hall of Australia Pty. Limited, *Sydney*
Prentice-Hall Canada Inc., *Toronto*
Prentice-Hall Hispanoamericana, S.A., *Mexico*
Prentice-Hall of India Private Limited, *New Delhi*
Prentice-Hall of Japan, Inc., *Tokyo*
Simon & Schuster Asia Pte. Ltd., *Singapore*
Editora Prentice-Hall do Brasil Ltda., *Rio de Janeiro*

Contents

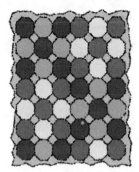

About the Authors

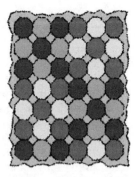

Michael Appleton grew up in Los Angeles, California. He attended UCLA premedical and graduated from the California College of Medicine, University of California-Irvine. He was trained in internal medicine at Los Angeles County Medical Center, and practiced in Burbank, California for thirty years.

Doctor Appleton has directed the intensive and cardiac care units at Thompson Memorial Medical Center in Burbank. A pivotal point in his thinking on dying occurred when he met and became friends with Elisabeth Kubler-Ross and assisted in her workshops on death, dying, and transition.

He's been the medical director of the Visiting Nurse Association of Los Angeles, Hospice in the Home, since 1984, and from this position makes about forty-five home visits each month to terminally ill patients who are enrolled in the hospice program. Doctor Appleton is also a frequent speaker and presenter at the National Hospice Organization.

Doctor Appleton wrote the section on hospice medicine for the "Merck Manual," and he is certified in addiction medicine by the American Society of Addiction Medicine.

When he has the time, he and his wife Susan, a psychotherapist, like to listen to jazz. Michael is also a professional bass player (his stepfather played bass in the Los Angeles Philharmonic), and when he has the time, he plays at a few Los Angeles jazz clubs. In 1994, he plans to relocate to Missoula, Montana.

Todd Henschell is a freelance writer and screenwriter, whose long association with Michael Appleton as both a patient and friend led to his involvement in this project. He has a B.S. degree in writing and psychology from Eastern Michigan University and a longstanding interest in technical and medical subjects. He has written for film and television and, along with having put words on paper about subjects ranging from automobiles to xenophobia, has a regular column in the national newspaper *Computer World.*

In his spare time he likes to tinker with his three computers, run with his Airedale Mad Max, and listen to classical music with his true love, Leslie. He hopes the last music to grace his ears will be Mahler's Ninth Symphony, Fourth Movement, the Adagio.

Authors' Note

Much of the information in this book is based upon my years of experience as a hospice physician. A lot of this book is my opinion. There is room for disagreement, and often new information makes what we now call "truth" into "untruth." This is the way of medical and scientific progress, which is—and should be—a dynamic and changing affair.

Where I was able to do so, I've given credit to those whose thoughts I've borrowed. If I've forgotten to mention someone, it was only because I couldn't remember the source, so I apologize to you and thank you.

Special thanks to all my friends, coworkers, and acquaintances who've contributed their ideas and impressions. This book would never have seen the light of day without them.

Above all, first and foremost, thanks to my wife Sue: my best friend and most loving critic.

M.A. October 1993

For my mother and Father, who have always had faith in me.

T.H. October 1993

A Family Guide To Dying At Home

Physicians usually don't have the chance to observe the slow transition from life to death as it occurs in patients who are dying at home. Hospice staff and volunteers spend more time with dying patients, and often are able to guide the family through the process of death.

All of us in hospice care try to reassure the patient and family as death approaches. Attending to a dying person can be physically and emotionally exhausting. It's tough, demanding work—but it also can be an extremely satisfying and rewarding experience. The time of closure is a chance for emotional wounds to heal and relationships to come full circle. It's a chance to say things never said. It's a time to say good-bye.

There is no "standard" way to die—no set path everybody follows. There are some common signs and symptoms that, if understood, make the process much easier. During this stressful period, caregivers may get complicated opinions from many sources. Because of the powerful emotions of the moment, some people can't absorb all the advice they receive from the medical professionals working with them. Caregivers worry about making mistakes. Most of this worry is unfounded. Your instincts are always your best guide.

This book is a practical reference. It's my way of sharing with you the things I've discovered during my practice that have helped those with whom I've worked. This book should help you understand the events that are natural to the end of life. It should relieve the nagging uncertainty, self-doubt, and the confusion that surrounds the events of dying. I hope it frees caregivers to function more smoothly and allows them to help the dying patient achieve more comfort.

As life ends, patients withdraw. They tend to eat and drink less and exhibit other visible changes from their "normal" behavior. Strong emotions may surface in the caregivers, taking them by surprise. These things are natural; none of them should be dreaded or feared. I'll try to describe some of the changes and problems in the pages that follow, and I'll relate some significant events that altered how I viewed death.

This book is divided into sections, by topic, and some subjects are cross-referenced and found under another topic. I guarantee that this book is incomplete. With any luck at all, I've managed to include the essentials. You should be able to look up signs or symptoms and find information that simplifies difficult situations.

The most frequent question caregivers ask me is: "How long do you think it will be?" Missing from the end of that question, hanging over it like the sword of legend, is "until the patient dies"? I never know for sure. I do know that the question is a reflection of the caregiver's need to talk, to be reassured by someone in authority, to know that things will work out. We need to know that things will be okay, that blazing pain and horrible symptoms can be managed. We need to be reassured that the patient will not die alone and that we will not be overwhelmed by it all and swallowed up by our emotions.

It's impossible to know precisely when the patient will die. A rough estimate and careful appreciation of the signposts along the way can help the caregiver plan and prepare for the final hour. Medical professionals who have seen death can sometimes seem aloof and distant. It's easy to forget that death is a once-in-a-lifetime event for the patient.

Death is a unique experience. It deserves our attention.

How to Use This Book

This book is designed to be "user-friendly." That means we tried to provide well-organized answers to your questions about what happens when people choose to die at home. We want the information and the suggestions to be of real practical value. We want to help you understand and cope with the powerful emotional and physical demands that will be put upon you at the end of a friend's or loved one's life.

Are you concerned about symptoms or the events that take place? Are you wondering if what you're going through is going the way it is "supposed" to be? We hope you'll be able to find a key word in the table of contents and turn to a page with some simple, understandable answers.

It's probably better if you read the book from cover to cover. I'm sure you'll recognize some familiar situations. I also hope that you'll learn some things that will make your journey easier. That we help you remains our most important goal.

Foreword

The genesis of any book is a mysterious experience. The genesis of *At Home with Terminal Illness*, by Michael Appleton, M.D. and Todd Henschell proves this point. Often we visit our doctor carrying a list of "Remembering to ask the doctor..." questions. Over his years of practice, Dr. Appleton was the recipient of many questions regarding terminal illness. Wanting to provide the answers, he took pen in hand and compiled this Family Guidebook to Hospice in the Home. I wish I had owned this book when, in 1979, I shared the last weeks of caregiving for my father who suffered inoperable colon cancer.

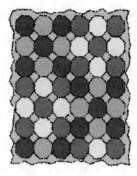

In *Proverbs 3:27–28* it says, "Do not withhold good from those to whom it is due, when it is in the power of your hand to do so."

At Home with Terminal Illness is such a "good." Dr. Appleton seeks to guide the nonprofessional caregiver who is emotionally involved in the task at hand. He knows they are accompanying a loved one on the last steps of the journey of life. This book will simplify the caregiver's search for information regarding terminal illness. Dr. Appleton and Mr. Henschell write in plain, simple English. There is no jargon or medical "codes" to baffle the layman.

As a Hospice Board Director, Trustee, and Volunteer I'm very proud and grateful for this book's contribution to the hospice movement. The authors' urging to *"add to the quality of the remaining days rather than simply adding days"* is moving and reassuring to the caregiver. Health care costs are rising, and we must embrace the hospice movement—and the simple, elegant nature of hospice itself—as a recognized medical option in caring for the terminally ill patient. No other system offers such compassionate care combined with prudent expense.

Death is the end of life. Our society needs to hear the authors' messages. If the reader takes these to heart, he or she will learn how to identify, accept, and react to the signs of death along the path. This book shows the way to adding quality to life—and it is quality, not quantity, that is our goal when helping the terminally ill. *Better* days, not *more* days, is the message here.

I thank Michael Appleton for remembering those anxious caregivers of the past. I thank him and Todd Henschell for preparing this text for those now caring for a dying loved one, and those in the future who will face this difficult task. The authors' professionalism, wisdom, humor, and sensitivity make this book a priceless gift for those who need it most. The caregiver who holds this guide has, in *At Home with Terminal Illness*, a friend who is ready to help in a time of need.

Sister Karen Burns

Acceptance

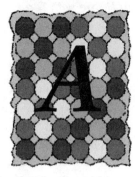

People frequently misunderstand the term "acceptance." It comes from Elisabeth Kubler-Ross's book *On Death and Dying*. She describes the emotional stages or coping mechanisms that we see in patients with terminal illness. Sometimes we think of acceptance as "giving up." This is inaccurate. Others look at acceptance as a goal the patient needs to reach—an end in itself—something all patients should strive toward. This, too, is wrong.

Not all patients can accept the reality of the end of their life. Many patients need to distance themselves from the process in which they're involved right to the end. It might be too painful to accept fully what's going on. Acceptance isn't *all or none*. There are degrees of acceptance. People may seem more accepting of dying and at peace at one moment and very resistant a bit later. Acceptance is an accommodation to reality. Some people can more deeply embrace reality than others.

Remember: *You should meet people where they* ***are****, not where you think they ought to be.*

Each person travels his or her path, not yours, and not mine. Sometimes it's hard to stay on the path, and much of "working through" happens at a subconscious level. It occurs at *whatever pace is appropriate for each individual.*

Acceptance means allowing things to be exactly as they are. That doesn't mean we have to like the situation, but it seems that the longer we resist things, the longer they persist, as if the resistance holds things in place.

Letting things go may be a lot easier said than done—and it doesn't happen all at once. Letting go, surrendering, and all those ways of relinquishing control represent a process. Fortunately, in hospice, we don't have to do it alone. We can let go of resistance in the company of those we love.

The "stages of dying" apply not only to the terminally ill patient—they also apply to family and friends. It's hard to accept that a friend and loved one is dying. It's also hard to admit that there is no cure, and some people equate lack of cure with "no hope."

In hospice we treat pain and symptoms. People sometimes ask: "What do you mean, nothing more can be done?" The plain truth is that life always reaches an end, and many ailments that affect us will advance to a point beyond cure—but we should never reach a point where we don't care. Patients and families often feel abandoned by their doctors who honestly say, "There's nothing more I can do." Actually, there's a lot more doctors can do. We can communicate that, even though there's no possible cure, we still *care*. And we can treat discomfort.

I was in an auto accident several years ago, saw many physicians, and had lots of tests. Not once did any doctor say, "I'm sorry you're having pain," or "This must be miserable for you." That sure would have made a world of difference to me. They did almost all the right medical things—except to express caring. That concern may be there in many doctors who reach the end of the curative road with their patients, but they often don't express it. It would certainly reduce the feeling of being abandoned if we really knew that our doctors cared. It could make acceptance a little easier.

When we feel a compulsion to "reclassify" a terminally ill person into a new stage (such as acceptance) or out of a stage (such as denial), we ought to examine if our motivation for worrying about such things is for the patient's good or to make ourselves more comfortable. Patients or caregivers can't go wrong if they remember and recite the Serenity Prayer:

> God grant me the serenity
> to accept the things I cannot change,
> the courage to change the things I can, and the
> wisdom to know the difference.

Agitation

Agitation at the end of life is difficult to manage. The combination of agitation and confusion is called *delirium*. Before the caregiver assumes that the patient's agitation is caused by underlying

2

disease, suspect drugs or a multiple-drug interaction—particularly suspicious are any new additions to the patients drug regimen. Drug interactions and drug-combined effects cause many behavioral disturbances. Stop giving the patient all nonessential drugs. Agents such as halloperidol (Haldol) can help a confused patient, and they won't produce sedation.

Make sure your physician monitors all the possible side effects of the medications administered to the patient.

Other things can cause the patient to become agitated. Look for a full bladder (and difficulty in emptying it), constipation, fecal impaction, severe pain, and itching. All these can be treated if you keep and eye out for them and recognize them. Watch out for signs of anxiety, fear, and other emotional reactions.

You should follow these steps:

1. Stop administering all nonessential drugs.
2. Look for other causes that can create discomfort.
3. If you can't find any physical difficulty, and you've tried everything you can, the only practical solution might be to use a drug such as Haldol. Always consult your doctor.

Don't discount the effects of music or of sitting with the patient to reduce the patient's feeling of isolation. Keep the room open and airy. A view of the outside, if that's available, is almost always a pleasant addition to the room and may calm some patients (as well as give them something to look at other than four boring walls or a babbling television).

Try to avoid using restraints unless the patient's behavior becomes violent and can cause harm to the patient or caregiver. If the patient needs to be restrained, try a Posey belt; it secures the body without tying down the arms.

Remember: *When we cannot cure: comfort always.*

AIDS

Why is AIDS (acquired immune deficiency syndrome) different from any other terminal illness? While AIDS is still a disease with no known cure, death from AIDS is usually caused by the opportunistic infections or tumors that attack the AIDS patient. Sometimes these can be treated and cured, but the underlying problem (the human immunodeficiency virus itself) can't be cured. There are medicines available to slow the HIV and prolong life, but they cannot yet cure the ailment.

Also, the image of AIDS for some people brings up strong negative feelings. They think of homosexuals, drug abusers, and contagious diseases and forget that it's a human being suffering beneath these unfavorable stereotypes. When we think of cancer we often see a poor victim—despite the fact that many cancers are self-inflicted, such as lung cancer from smoking. When we think of AIDS, sadly, we often seem to lose our sympathy, and many people have this hidden voice saying, "They asked for it." Well, they didn't, and this is an improper approach to caring for any patient.

AIDS commonly affects young people, and—understandably—they're reluctant to enter hospice while there is "hope" that they will be able to recover. They may view hospice as giving up, and that can be a horrible recognition for them. This can create powerful and complex emotions with which they'll have to cope, adding more stress to the physical stress the syndrome causes.

One of the problems with AIDS is that, while it's presently a terminal illness, it isn't *immediately terminal*. This means that often patients with HIV are reluctant to enter a hospice when there are treatments for the infections that, untreated, used to cause death. Given that hospice is dedicated to neither hastening death nor prolonging the process of dying, does this mean that HIV-infected patients can't be in a hospice program if they are on "curative" drugs? Does this mean that AIDS patients must forsake all these kinds of drugs to qualify for hospice?

These are difficult decisions we must make about the treatment of HIV patients in hospice. Each patient's case is different, and should be considered unique. In some cases, hospice rules will need to be changed. New drugs are being developed and introduced, and these can alter the prognosis and the nature of hope. There are also patients who aren't benefiting from treatment, and for them, the decision to enter hospice is appropriate.

Because of the stigma of AIDS, the cost of care and factors affecting health insurance, many AIDS patients don't have access to solid mainstream medical care. This is an embarrassing tragedy in our society.

Allergy

People may claim to be allergic to medication when they're simply suffering from the side effects of a drug. Certain antibiotics produce intestinal upset because they alter the normal bacterial populations in the gut. This isn't an allergy. Patients who have previously had problems with opiates such as codeine or morphine often confuse side effects with allergy and refuse to take a valuable medication.

True allergy usually causes hives (large irregular reddish raised and itchy welts). True morphine allergy is extremely rare. And if the patient takes drugs such as morphine for awhile, most side effects may lessen or even disappear.

Alternative Medicine?

I prefer the term *adjunctive* medicine, since *alternative* medicine suggests abandoning conventional therapy in favor of another healing method.

There are many ways of healing that aren't universally accepted. Although there may be no "scientific" explanation for them, they work. The big question is whether these techniques are really effective—or do they work because of the placebo effect? All this is open to debate, and we don't have enough space to work that subject to a proper conclusion here—it's not the purpose of this book. If these nonstandard techniques help the person *feel better* and don't cause injury or interfere with effective treatments, we can certainly accept them. We should even consider them valuable, because the placebo effect alone is powerful and beneficial.

People disillusioned with the limitations of mainstream medicine often look for hope elsewhere. It's an easy market ripe with desperate patients, and where there are gaps in traditional medicine—and these gaps do exist—there are always people willing to offer hope and miracles. Sometimes these practitioners are fast-buck artists, and other times they deeply believe in the kind of healing they practice.

In years past, hypnosis, visual imagery, acupuncture, and manipulative therapy were frowned upon, even considered quackery. Today there's room for these techniques alongside—not in place of—established treatment.

There are exceptions to every rule, and while we see now how important good diet is, how essential proper nutrition is to health, special "toxic cleansing" diets, herbal concoctions, and tortuous colonic treatments may weaken sick people. This makes them harmful, and thus something to avoid. Consider how a healthy person might react to severe routines such as these, subtract half or more of that person's stamina, and look at it again. Stay away from unnecessary things that are hurtful. Remember, the patient's days are, by definition, limited. We don't want to add any more hurt than absolutely necessary.

A problem with all of medicine is the tendency of the parties involved to get so absorbed in the treatment that neither caregiver nor patient can recognize that the process isn't working. The treatment becomes an end in itself, and everyone involved forgets the real goal, which is to make the patient feel better. Many practitioners of alternative medicine genuinely care about their patients, and some are, as I said, in it for the money. Others mean well, but are poorly trained, ill-informed, or inexperienced with certain ailments.

When aggressive therapy is pursued for therapy's sake—or profit—the patient is going to get lost in the shuffle. Stressful treatments take away precious "quality time" from the person with incurable illness. Time is the most precious thing a terminally ill person has.

I remember Shannon…

She was a courageous and defiant young woman who discovered a mass in her right breast. She hoped it would go away. It didn't. As the mass grew larger, she was fearful and embarrassed that she'd let it go for so long.

When she finally saw a physician, he did a biopsy and told her that she had breast cancer. He then berated her for not seeking treatment sooner (as if that would help her now). During a social visit with me she placed my hand on her breast and asked me what I thought. I must've looked shocked—judging by her reaction. I told her that it needed to be treated soon.

Instead, she chose to see a spiritual healer who advised a cure with a macrobiotic diet and prolonged meditation. She didn't improve. Perhaps she even felt as if she were a failure—if she had only done enough, it would've worked.

She went to the East Coast for surgery and chemotherapy at a large medical center. This provided only a brief period of remission from this aggressive tumor. She decided to abandon any further conventional treatment and went, instead, to a Mexican clinic for a program of fasting and enemas. She became so weak that she had to be brought home by ambulance. Hospice in the home cared for her until her death.

People told me that I shouldn't be upset—that I shouldn't have such an investment in my kind of treatment. People said, "That was the way she had to do it," and "It was her way." But I was disappointed. I had envisioned a smoother course that would have added comfort, as well as quality time, to her life.

What would I have done in a similar situation? I think that I would have chosen a more conventional treatment. I would have also used as many "adjunctive" treatments as possible, if I thought they might help. I would have steered clear of healers who condemned conventional therapy, and those who advised that I "throw out the baby with the bath water."

I'd be just as skeptical of mainstream doctors who automatically condemned all forms of alternate medicine, or who patronized me. Above all, I know that I'd search out someone I could trust, someone whose honesty and integrity I felt with my heart. I would leave my fate in that person's hands and work with them.

Not everybody needs to do it my way.

The mission of hospice is to add *more life to the patient's days*— not necessarily more days to his or her life.

Alternatives to Dying at Home

Most people would prefer to die at home. There is the family, familiar surroundings, and the collection of things we love that comedian George Carlin calls "our stuff." We are set at ease when we have *our stuff* at hand. It's simple enough, but it's an important thing to remember.

Caring for a dying person can be physically and emotionally exhausting. Sometimes the patient's pain and symptoms can't be managed at home, despite the best efforts of family and friends. A hospital, skilled nursing facility, or a hospice inpatient facility might be a better choice if the patient's quality of life suffers at home.

Sometimes caregivers feel guilty, as if they were derelict in their duties because they weren't able to keep the patient at home. Perhaps the patient was insistent that he or she stay at home, and when this isn't a practical solution, the person caring for them feels like a failure. They weren't able to fulfill this very important wish. Things are rarely that simple, and turning the patient over to the hands of an experienced professional may be best choice.

Once treated by professionals, the patient might rest easier, and the caregiver will have some time to recover, as well. Finally, it should allow both patient and caregiver a breather, giving both of them more quality time to share at the end. Discuss these decisions openly with family and friends.

Anger

Anger isn't usually considered a primary emotion. In some ways, anger and depression are related. Depression can be anger turned inward. When a person is unable to change his situation to his liking, anger or depression is often the result. Anger is the expression of unhappiness with the way things are.

Anger is sometimes a substitute for feelings that the patient can't express easily, such as sadness, embarrassment, fear, or ill-defined feelings of loss. Anger is difficult to tolerate when it's directed at us. A witness to anger is also the victim of anger, and may feel personally attacked, even if the anger is directed at another target.

Remember: *Try not to take anger personally.*

One problem with anger is that it alienates people, pushing away the comfort and help a caregiver can provide. Those who feel alone and isolated will find these feelings aggravated by their tantrums and hostile comments. If you keep this in mind, and realize that anger is often a reflection of pain, you'll be able to help the patient work through these feelings. This will reduce the patient's anger, eventually, and minimize the amount of stress everybody else has to weather.

> Anger must come from judgment. Judgment is the weapon I would use against myself, to keep the miracle away from me.
> —Helen Schucman, William Thetford, *A Course in Miracles*, © 1983, Foundation for Inner Peace.

Anxiety

Anxiety is a state of uneasiness or apprehension. Situations about which patients or families feel anxious can be real or imagined, but the feeling—and the resulting stress—is very real. It's important to reassure and comfort the patient when anxiety becomes a problem. When this isn't enough, tranquilizers may be required. The best tranquilizers are the short-acting benzodiazepines such as Ativan. Long-acting drugs can remain in the body too long, causing extended drowsiness. The caregiver might not want to sedate a dying patient, and that's understandable.

Remember, though, that the main goal should always be the patient's comfort. Excess sedation may be a necessary trade-off.

Anxiety can be caused by the patient's fear about the end of life, the loss of control, the fear of pain or other concerns. Allowing a patient to talk about these fears can help. Other patients may fear pain, suffocation, choking, bleeding, and other problems they may have or fear they might develop. In these cases, the reassurance of a hospice professional is required. Patients may have seen or heard about a horrible death caused by the same disease they themselves have.

Talk to the patient. Support their concerns. Reassurance is essential.

Remember: *Do not minimize, dismiss, or patronize—anxiety is **real**.*

Attitude

Exchanging pleasantries at social events usually includes the question, "What do you do?" When people ask me, I'm tempted to say, "The Good Work," but I don't. I'm also tempted to lie, and claim to be an accountant, something that can easily be passed over so we can move on to a discussion of sports or the weather. If I say I'm a physician, I'm usually asked what kind, and when I state that I'm an internist, the next question is: "What specialty?" So I usually just come out and say that I am a hospice physician. Following a brief pause, which occasionally includes an uncomfortable *gulp*, comes the standard response, "Oh my, that must be depressing." *Attitude...*

Some people don't know what hospice is, so when I explain that I take care of people who are dying, I get a reply like: "Why the hell would you pick that line of work?" *Attitude...*

Rarely do people say, "Why how interesting, tell me more about it." I even had a colleague say, "Tell me about your hospice work, but just leave out that dying stuff." Physicians usually have some opinions about hospice—that it's advanced hand-holding, or skilled pastoral care, or some fringe group where patients should be referred when there's nothing more to do. *Attitude...*

Some physicians avoid hospice like a plague while holding on to the myth that hospice is less scientific, or is euthanasia in camouflage. *Attitude...* Many physicians now accept hospice as part of mainstream medicine.

When patients and their families tell us how wonderful our hospice program is, and that they don't know how they would have survived without it, they frequently add: "Why didn't we know about you sooner?" *Attitude...*

People don't want to talk about dying until it hits them in the face. Why should they? Many physicians think of referring patients to hospice as a sign of failure or giving up. *More attitude.*

Most of you who will read this book already know about hospice and the care of terminal illness—you will likely have experienced some part of it or you wouldn't be reading the book. You might even have had a positive experience caring for a dying person. Perhaps these words are like a church sermon. The people in church aren't the ones who need to hear the sermon; it's the folks outside who should hear it. Anyway, I'd like to take a moment to share my attitude. I have one, too.

I think hospice medicine is a wonderful specialty. It's real family medicine, and it treats the entire person, the physical, social, emotional, and spiritual.

Hospice people are dedicated and courageous. They make a contribution to the lives of the dying, knowing full well that they will lose *all* their patients. Yet they are willing to accept the fact that they will eventually suffer a loss. It's difficult for people who aren't involved with hospice to realize just how rewarding this work is. It's rewarding precisely because we have an attitude.

We believe that each moment of life counts. We try to live our life that way and help others cherish life. We realize that we can't win, but we try to make the loss as graceful and dignified as possible.

We have a very self-serving attitude that comes from the experience of getting more in the long run than we give.

We have the attitude that our lives are immeasurably enriched by our work, and by the difference we make in the lives of others.

Baldness

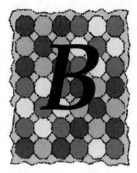

Hair loss can be caused because of radiation therapy or chemotherapy. Irregular hair loss may leave the scalp looking moth-eaten and ragged. It doesn't look the same as male pattern baldness. Usually patients are warned about this side effect. Nevertheless, it's shocking to see a person who has suddenly lost a full head of hair. The patient's self-image may suffer, compounding any other problems he or she is having. When a patient's hair does fall out, it's likely to be distressing. In our culture we worry quite a bit about how we look, and suddenly finding yourself bald isn't a choice experience. This is even more stressful for women patients, in some cases. When the hair does return, it might be darker, more coarse, or even curly where it was straight before.

Wigs and caps can help reduce the self-consciousness of the patient whose hair has fallen out.

One of my patients a few years ago was a handsome man with a thick head of hair. While undergoing chemotherapy for leukemia, he lost his hair. He refused to allow any visitors to see him because he was embarrassed by how he looked. When a group of his men friends found out about his baldness, they came up with a solution: they all had their heads shaved and then went together to visit him at the hospital.

When the patient saw that his buddies were bald, too, the group shared a good laugh about how they all looked. The patient realized that his baldness certainly wasn't the major problem he'd thought it to be.

Bargaining

Bargaining is one way that we attempt to deal with a threat to our *self*. Elisabeth Kubler-Ross discusses this as an ego-coping mechanism in her book *On Death and Dying*.

Bargaining is a kind of wishful thinking—in dying patients, it represents hope. The person wants to strike a deal just to get an extra bit of life in trade for something else. The problem is: What's to trade and who can grant the request?

Children sometimes think this way: "I promise that I will be good and do the thing you want me to do, if only...."

Bargaining is a way of working things out, a stalling technique that buys time while the person sorts through options. It's the *Maybe-ifs*, a kind of internal procrastination of the mind, and the main purpose it serves is to buy escape time from dealing with the hard reality of oncoming death.

The simple fact that bargaining happens indicates some degree of acceptance (of death), but it also illustrates that the patient hasn't relinquished all hope.

Bedsores

Bedsores (decubiti) are ulcers that result from pressure against the skin. Other factors can contribute to their development and aggravate them. Poor nutrition, lack of good blood flow to the skin, and constant rubbing and shearing forces (sliding across the bed) all come into play in producing bedsores.

Bedsores are graded from 1 to 4 depending on their depth. They usually occur on the backside, but they're not limited to that location. Anywhere there is skin a bedsore can develop. Most of the time they're present over bony areas, and on skin where body fat used to be. Turning the patient frequently helps to prevent bedsores, because no one area is under steady pressure for too long. Special mattresses such as egg-crate or alternating-pressure air cushions can help. In some cases, the patient is so emaciated and blood circulation is so poor that bedsores develop despite the caregiver's best efforts. The appearance of bedsores isn't always a sign of poor care or negligence.

There are many treatments for bedsores. Most of all, remember that they're painful, and that treatment of terminal illness requires relief from all pain. Bedsores are no exception.

Sometimes when I make a home visit, I won't attempt to turn the patient during the examination because I want to avoid causing pain. Since I haven't looked at the patient's backside, I ask the caregivers if there are any bedsores. If there are none, the caregivers usually respond with a strong, "No!" They're proud of the fact. Sometimes they follow this with a look that asks: *How could you think such a thing*?

When the caregivers have to say, "Yes," they usually make an attempt to explain, such as "He came home from the hospital that way." If the patient has bedsores, we immediately think he or she has been neglected and that the caregivers have been negligent. The fact is, despite the best care, bedsores can be impossible to prevent. Patients will frequently find a comfortable position and refuse to move out of it, increasing the chance that bedsores will develop.

Bereavement

Bereavement isn't a "state," it's a process. It's the process of recovering, of healing—both emotionally and physically—from the death of a loved one. This can take a long time, sometimes several years. There is no specific date when you are supposed to "get over" the loss and get "back to business." Many people find professional counseling helps during this period. Suffering alone and "toughing it out" is an outmoded idea. It belongs with "willpower" and "keeping a stiff upper lip." Getting help in a time of emotional crisis is a much better than experiencing unnecessary and often prolonged suffering.

To love someone is to have that person be a reflection of the things you love about yourself. To love is to have part of yourself invested in the other person. To lose someone dear to us is painful and requires time to heal the wound left when "a piece of us dies."

Remember: *The essence of the healing process during bereavement is forgiveness.*

We must express our emotions for others to understand clearly what we are feeling. We must forgive a world where an event such as death can take our loved one away. We must forgive the medical professionals who sometimes appear uninterested and uncaring about our feelings. We must forgive those people who—for whatever reasons—were not there to support us when we needed them. We must forgive the dying person for leaving and abandoning us. We must forgive God for taking our loved one away and allowing bad things to happen to good people. Most of all, we must forgive ourselves for our failings and imperfections. We are, after all, only human.

Sometimes after the death of a loved one we think of things that we should have said or done. Obviously we can't do those things now. It's often helpful to write a letter to the person who has died and read it aloud as if they were listening. This can be an opportunity to express our feelings and set matters to rest.

Forgiveness isn't mandatory. We can continue to hold grudges, remain angry, and be legitimately self-righteous. This is a massive burden to carry, though, and eventually it will hurt the person struggling under it. Life and death are *not* fair, but forgiveness lightens the load and allows us to emerge from the shadow of death, back into life…that will continue with or without our participation.

Bone

Being inactive decreases the calcium content in bone, and the general strength of the skeleton deteriorates. Bone is more brittle in older people, and tumors (they often spread into bone) can further weaken the skeleton. Fractures in the ribs, long bones, and vertebrae accompany certain cancers. These injuries happen sometimes just by turning over in bed, and may not represent direct trauma. The bones are simply so fragile that normal motion can injure them.

In patients expected to recover, conventional care of fractures is appropriate. In terminally ill patients, the stress of surgery may outweigh the disadvantages of conservative care. Fractures normally placed in a cast can be splinted instead. Hip fractures, usually pinned in a surgical procedure, can be immobilized by "sandbagging" the patient into a comfortable position. The goal of fracture treatment here should always be to provide the most comfort and quality of life.

Surgery to treat a fracture shouldn't be performed simply because it's available, but surgery may be necessary to stabilize certain fractures. Bone pain can be relieved with aspirin or non-steroidal drugs such as ibuprofen (trade names are Motrin and Advil). If the patient has a hard time swallowing pills, there are liquid counterparts to the drugs just listed. Steroids such as prednisone also help bone pain. Although steroids do have some serious side effects over time, you shouldn't be as concerned about this when dealing with terminal illness. Some of the side effects are beneficial, such as increased appetite and a sense of well-being.

You can effectively relieve pain caused by cancer spreading into the bone with radiation therapy. The relief isn't immediate, and there may be a lot of discomfort (both physical and financial) in moving a person to and from the hospital or office to get treatment.

If the benefits don't outweigh the risks and discomfort, simpler treatment with medication may be the best.

Early one morning I arrived at a patient's home just as he was being moved on a stretcher by ambulance attendants. They were taking him for his prescribed radiation treatment. While X-ray therapy might've been the right thing to do for his disease, it wasn't the right thing to do for *him*. He was in a coma, and continuing treatment with radiation just wasn't appropriate. The attendants had their orders and proceeded to pack the patient into the ambulance and haul him away.

He died during the trip.

Bowels

Refer to the section on constipation.

Breathing

Breathing changes become more apparent as the end of life approaches. Oxygen can help relieve shortness of breath. You should provide it based on the patient's visible need, and a blood gas measurement isn't required. To determine if oxygen is helpful, simply watch to see if it makes the patient breath easier. If it does, then use it.

You will sometimes see irregular breathing, where the patient has periods of rapid and then slow breathing. This is called Chenye-Stokes breathing and shouldn't be harmful. Some patients may actually stop breathing for a few seconds. Usually breathing will start again, and the cycle will repeat.

Suctioning the airway if secretions have accumulated can relieve some breathing difficulties. Having the patient sit (if possible or practical) may make breathing easier, since it allows the patient's chest to expand more fully. Pain can cause breathing problems. Rib fractures, pleurisy, abdominal pain—any pain that is worsened by the motions of breathing—can be relieved with morphine or other opiates.

It's frightening for the patient who cannot breathe, or who imagines that he or she isn't getting enough air. Wheezing (the restriction of outward airflow) may accompany a tumor of the airway, congestive heart failure, asthma, or emphysema and requires prompt attention.

Burning

The sensation of burning can occur anywhere in the body. Burning indicates that nerves are being stimulated by inflammation or pressure. Burning in the skin may be caused by infections, such as shingles (herpes zoster), or might involve nerve cells directly, as in neuritis. Actual pressure on nerves from a tumor can cause burning pain. Tricyclic agents, often used to treat depression, can provide relief. If the patient's eyes are dry, they might burn, as well. Lubricating drops often help. Burning mouth can be caused by a vitamin deficiency or oral thrush (monilia). Antifungal mouth washes, gargles, and troches should help. Herpes may cause rectal burning. Vaginal and urethral burning are both quite common, and soothing lotions combined with topical anesthetics should prove useful.

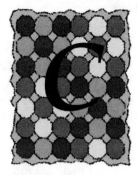

Cancer

Cancer is an ominous term that conjures up some very dark, very strong fears. For most patients, even *hearing* the word can imply the worst. The horoscope has abandoned the term in favor of "moon children." Because the word "cancer" is equated with death in the minds of most people, they often use less specific words, such as "tumor," "mass," "growth," "neoplasm," "spot," "lesion," and so on. *Cancer* is an appropriate term, and we should use it and deal with it without hesitation. Whispering the word indicates our discomfort.

While it's difficult to accept that cancer means a growth of a new kind of tissue within our body, and while it is a complicated and serious disease that takes many forms, we needn't hide from the fact that it *does* exist—whether we like it or not.

There are treatments for cancer, and when a cure isn't possible, therapy can be effective in retarding growth and improving the patient's health. Patients need to understand the extent of their disease and any potential for improvement. This includes describing any side effects that might happen because of the proposed therapy. Not all symptoms that occur in cancer patients are due to the malignancy. We shouldn't assume that the cancer has caused the symptom and leave it at that *because the patient has cancer.* Evaluate and explain symptoms, don't just dismiss them as all being caused by the cancer itself.

Physicians should have a frank discussion of the disease with the patient, explain the various options available, and the likely consequences of decisions either way. Respecting the patient's right to make this choice (it is the *patient's* life we're talking about) is important.

Some patients choose to avoid talking about their disease. A woman once told me that she had "a little cancer." That meant to me that she had " a little denial" about the extent of her disease. Some people prefer to avoid discussing cancer and change the subject, while others forge ahead, determined to "beat it."

It isn't necessary for patients to deal with their concerns about cancer alone. It helps to get involved with cancer support groups where patients and their families can openly discuss their feelings and get help sorting things out.

Catheters

Many patients with terminal illness lose control of their bowels and bladder. Lying in wet bedclothes and having continually wet garments can cause the tissues in the groin to become water-logged and break down. This can cause inflammation and pain. Although urinary catheters aren't ideal (they frequently lead to urinary infections), the trade-off might be necessary to increase comfort. A patient who can't pass urine also might require a catheter. (Inability to urinate can be caused by physical obstruction of the tract, spinal cord compression by a tumor, or ingestion of certain medications.)

Certain antihistamines, tranquilizers, and antidepressants can cause urinary difficulty. In these cases, a catheter might not be required if you stop administering the offending drug. A catheter can diminish the embarrassment the patient might feel at having to wear a diaper. The catheter should always be taped to the patient's leg to avoid pulling on the bladder and urethra.

I examined a woman recently who suddenly became unable to urinate. Her bladder was enlarged, and I could easily feel it during my examination. She also developed weakness in her legs, and a saddlelike area became numb. She was suffering from spinal cord compression due to a tumor. She required a catheter immediately to drain her bladder. But more important, we had to make a decision about how to treat the spinal cord compression that was causing her problem.

Had this happened early in her illness, we would have prescribed radiation therapy to shrink the tumor and limit or prevent her paralysis. Sometimes we use large doses of steroids first, because if that helps, it's a sign that radiation should help, too.

In this particular situation, the patient's disease was very far advanced, and resorting to putting her in the hospital and having her undergo radiation therapy, would have severely compromised her fragile state. I went over the options with the family (she was too weak to participate), and we decided to do as much as possible to provide immediate comfort in the home.

When sudden changes such as this happen, the hospice nurse of physician should be notified *immediately*. Only then can the family and the medical professionals come to the correct decision on treatment.

Chemotherapy

Chemotherapy is a general term that refers to the drugs (which are chemicals) used to treat cancer. Treatment might be a single drug, or a combination of drugs, depending upon the malignancy cell type and its stage of growth. The duration of "chemo" courses vary, and have different outcomes. Most cancers can't be completely cured, but many do respond to treatment. The result of therapy may be improvement or a remission with an increased life span. It isn't possible to predict how every treatment will work, and the patient might need a therapeutic trial.

Most forms of chemotherapy have side effects. The chemical agents used in therapy interrupt cellular functioning. Although they're more active against cancer cells, they affect normal cells, too. Weakness, loss of hair, vomiting, and diarrhea are just a few of the undesirable side effects. Depression of bone marrow cells can produce anemia, lower the white blood cell count, and make the patient prone to infection. The ability of the patient's blood to clot normally can also suffer. The decision to use chemotherapy requires weighing the benefits against the risks. Obviously, chemotherapy shouldn't be chosen simply because it's available and offers "something to do."

If "chemo" allows a patient to live longer with a life that's comfortable and worthwhile, then it's appropriate. If the side effects are likely to make the patient miserable and diminish the quality of life, then it's best withheld. Sometimes it's simply impossible to predict the response, and chemotherapy is offered as a "window of hope." Ask yourself: "How large is that window?" and "How does it compare to doing nothing?" When chemotherapy is offered as a way to make us better, ask: *Will I feel better? How long will it be until I feel better? How much better do you think I'll feel? And for how long will feeling better last?*

These are tough questions. There may be no exact answers.

It is important to ask them, however, and to listen carefully to the advice of professionals. Listen to *everything* that's said, not just what you find hopeful and comfortable to hear. Other opinions might help to digest the options for the cancer patient. We must trust the physicians in whose hands we place our lives. Don't be guided by fear, but don't rely on mere hopes and dreams to guide you. Trust your intuition.

Understand that even when you've done all the necessary investigation, asked all the "right" questions, and followed your best judgments, things may still go awry. Don't bemoan the fact that things didn't go as well as they should have.
Life is what happens to us after we've made plans.

In hospice, where the goal is a palliative treatment (to make the patient feel better) and not "cure," chemotherapy has little place. Remember, again, that the intention of hospice is to add more life to one's days, not more days to one's life.

Children

Because my experience in caring for children with terminal illness is limited, I won't attempt to discuss in detail the topic of dying children. What I have seen of it tells me that children who are dying are often less fearful than their parents, and are also able to understand the severity of their illness. If you want to read more about this, there are several excellent texts available through the American Cancer Society and the National Hospice Organization.

I feel children should be included in—and not excluded from—the process of dying in the home (or hospital). Excluding children from participating prevents them from experiencing closure (which they will do in their own way), and it perpetuates the myth that there's something unacceptable and frightening about the end of life. Children who participate in the death of a family

21

member feel useful, important, and respected. They stand a better chance of becoming adults without developing a morbid fear of dying.

Children also have a wonderfully open way of dealing with a terminally ill family member, and their participation can enhance the quality of life of the dying person. The comfort and joy from a cheerfully unaffected child can be much more pleasurable than the well-meaning and appropriately somber adult.

On one home visit a 5-year-old girl answered the door. I told her I was the doctor, and she led me by the hand. "Come with me," she said, "I'll take you to my Grandma. You know she's dying, don't you?"

On a related subject, try not to use the word sleep when explaining death to children. Such phrases as, "We put the dog to sleep," may frighten children. They may equate going to bed (and sleeping) with dying. Healthy people awaken from sleep. Dying people may sleep and then die.

Whenever we lose someone or something that we love, we lose the piece of ourselves that we have invested in that relationship. Grief is the expression of our loss, and the period of healing is bereavement. When children die, the loss seems far greater. There is lost potential. We invest in our children the hopes and dreams that may not have been fulfilled in our lifetime.

Our children represent us—in fact they are us, genetically speaking. To lose a child is to lose a real part of us—the genes that went into making our child. There's also a common belief that we are responsible for our children, and we need to protect them from harm until they are old enough and big enough to take care of themselves. When a child dies, a part of us can feel as if we didn't provide that protection.

Color

The terminally ill patient's skin or nailbeds often change color. Lack of oxygen can give the skin and lips a bluish hue. The nails might appear purple (a sign of cyanosis). Jaundice is a yellow stain in the skin that's caused by an accumulation of bile. This happens when there are problems with the liver and bile can't drain normally into the intestine. When this occurs, bowel movements are usually colorless. Anemic patients can appear pale and washed-out. Some patients with respiratory failure can look flushed. Don't let color changes alarm you, and worse yet, don't let them prevent you from physical contact with the patient. Our need for a kind touch doesn't diminish when we are terminally ill.

Colostomy

A stoma is an opening. A colostomy is an opening from the colon (large intestine) to the outside of the body. The patient or caregiver places a bag over the opening to collect the fecal contents of the colon that pass from the large intestine. Obstruction of the colon, usually by cancer, may require only a resection (removing a part and connecting the remaining parts). Many times the surgeon performing the colostomy has to divert the colon to the outside of the body, because the malignancy has involved too much tissue to repair it.

Whatever the reason for this surgery, it can allow patients to function and continue meaningful lives with minimal discomfort and inconvenience. It's essential to learn about colostomy care, and I suggest you obtain the services of an expert, such as an eterostomal nurse. (This also applies to other ostomies such as ileostomy.)

Coma

Coma is a state of deep central nervous system depression. The patient may breathe and have a pulse, but isn't responsive to visual stimulation. Breathing can be slow and shallow. Patients with terminal illness don't usually awaken from coma. Many things can cause a comatose state, but drawn-out diagnostic studies and treatment are generally useless; treatment, in many cases, may only prolong dying.

Although we assume that comatose patients don't feel pain and are unable to hear, it can't hurt to continue talking to the patient—even if there is no response. Sometimes communication—

or an attempt at it—can be as helpful for the caregiver as it is for the one who is dying.

Confusion

Many terminally ill patients become confused. Their thinking becomes ill focused, and dying may worsen confusion that was already present, particularly in elderly patients. Poor blood flow to the brain, low oxygen and hemoglobin, metabolic problems (such as uremia from kidney failure), and complex interactions between medications are some of the causes. Keeping the room dark and whispering doesn't help dying persons with confused thoughts.

It's better to keep the room lighted, and the surroundings cheerful. It's much easier to focus on something you can see and hear. Talk to the patient in a normal voice. Touching and reassurance will help lessen confusion, also. If the patient is confused, take the time to answer the questions he or she might have. Suppress the urge to "humor" a confused person.

Confusion and disorientation can be frightening. Reassure and comfort the patient. It can be very difficult for the caregiver to manage a patient who has become confused, uncooperative, or even combatant. Even so, try to avoid using physical restraints. Chemical "restraints" such as sedatives or antianxiety drugs are better than tying the patient to the bed. Antipsychotic drugs can calm patients who are violent or combative. But first—before resorting to drugs (or finally) any type of physical restraint, check a few things:

1. If the patient has a catheter, is it plugged? Does the patient have a fecal impaction, a distended bladder, or some other uncomfortable problem that he or she can't communicate?

2. Is the patient on too many medications? Multiple drugs can interact with each other, producing toxic effects. Many drugs become toxic even with the "usual dose" if the patient is frail or unable to excrete the drug normally. Physicians sometimes prescribe a drug for each symptom without paying attention to how much other medicine patients have on board. The

next thing you know, the patient has problems caused by the treatment, not the original disease.

Specific medications, including oxygen, might help, and the caregiver should discuss them with the doctor or hospice nurse. The patient might improve if some medications were no longer administered. If a medicine is not *absolutely necessary*—if you can leave it out—do so. With terminally ill patients, the fewer medicines the better.

When in doubt, leave it out! But check with a professional first.

Congestion

There are many causes of congestion, one of which is administering intravenous fluids. The body may be unable to handle the usual amount of fluid, and attempts to "hydrate" a dying patient can worsen congestion. When you hear congestion in the upper airway, it's called the "death rattle." This is an unfortunate and grisly term.

These secretions can be difficult to cough up and hard to remove with suction. Medications such as atropine and scopolamine can reduce the secretions. Actually, the death rattle might be more unnerving for the people listening to it than the patient experiencing it.

Constipation

Constipation is the rule rather than the exception. Almost all patients immobilized in bed will become constipated. Altered diet and the use of medications—particularly morphine—contribute to the problem. You must routinely administer laxatives and enemas and pay attention to the patient's bowels to ensure the patient's comfort. Fecal impactions (the accumulation of hardened feces obstructing the lower colon) can be extremely uncomfortable.

The hospice nurse should frequently examine patients to detect an impaction while it is in an early stage. If one is present, it must be manually removed and prevented from recurring, if possible. Diarrhea may occasionally occur around a fecal impaction, and this can be a warning flag. For most people, their bowel habits have been a private (and potentially embarrassing) matter during adulthood.

Make whatever efforts are needed to ensure privacy and avoid embarrassment. It's essential to respect the patient's right to privacy while providing care.

Control

When I first started my work in hospice I found it curious that so many patients expected me to be punctual in my visits to their homes. They kept precise lists of medications and activities, and were generally demanding of their caregivers. It's the patient's need for control—or at least the illusion of control—that drove this behavior. People who were insecure and demanding and needed a rigid structure to their lives before their illness are often even more so when faced with dying.

For many people, dying is frightening. We lose much of the control we had in life, we can't do the things we want to do, and even some private functions (such as personal hygiene) have to be turned over to somebody else, sometimes a stranger. Both patients and caregivers attempt to exert influence over events that seem disorderly and unmanageable. Patients can appear fussy, unreasonable, and easily irritated when things are in disarray.

Try to understand the fear of losing control that underlies such behavior. Talk about these issues with the patient, or at least bring them up and make an effort to discuss them. It's helpful to allow and encourage as many activities as possible that will give the patient a sense of purpose and structure, and let them hold power over their fate.

When people are sick, particularly our loved ones, it's natural for us to want to do things for them to help make life easier. In doing so, we can contribute to their feelings of powerlessness and loss of control. Empowering people contributes to their sense of self-worth as human beings.

Remember: *Enabling patients to retain control is empowering and healing.*

To be alive is power,
Existing in itself,
Without further function,
Omnipotence enough.
                    —Emily Dickinson (Untitled poem no. 677)

Cough

Cough is a protective mechanism by which the airways expel an
irritant. A productive cough shouldn't be suppressed unless it's
preventing a patient from resting. Some coughs are dry and irritating. They also can be painful, and you should try to suppress
painful coughs. The best cough medications contain narcotics,
such as codeine and morphine. Use them as needed to ensure the
patient's comfort and rest.

Cramps

Cramps are painful involuntary muscle contractions. We call
intestinal cramps colic. These are recurring abdominal pains that
the patient feels as a tight, squeezing sensation in the gut. Sometimes intestinal cramping isn't associated with diarrhea, and
administering medication such as morphine can make it worse.
Atropine or scopolamine can help this type of cramping.

Bowel obstruction can also cause cramping. When the patient
is nauseous and vomiting, or suffers from abdominal distension,
his or her bowel might be obstructed. Conventional therapy is to
place a thin tube through the nose and down the alimentary canal,
into the stomach. Treatment of bowel obstruction can also involve
intravenous fluids and exploratory abdominal surgery.

In the hospice setting, the patient's weakened condition may
preclude surgery. Nasogastric tubes and intravenous fluids can
cause further discomfort and prolong the process of dying. The
treatment that offers the best quality of life—with the least pain
and suffering—is the treatment the caregiver should choose.

Cramps in the leg muscles can cause sudden pain and awak-
en patients at night. The patient can take benadryl or quinine prior
to sleep to prevent these muscle spasms.

Leg cramps can occur in healthy people as well as dying patients. Exercise-induced cramping and pain is called claudication and usually goes away with rest. It's due to poor circulation through tissues from narrowed blood vessels. Rest cramps aren't always easily explained. They may be caused by sudden changes in blood calcium, potassium, or sodium levels. Diuretics can sometimes cause rest cramps (probably from changing the levels of these electrolytes).

Crying

During my visits to hospice patients I hear their caregivers say such things as, "I don't want her to see me cry," or "I don't want to upset him." Why not cry? Crying is an expression of deep feeling. It's an indication of how strongly we feel about the loss of one whom we love. Such comments as "I don't want to get too emotional" suggest that there's a limit beyond which we shouldn't express feelings.

This idea is part of the old myths that "real men don't cry" and that suffering in silence with a stiff upper lip is somehow beneficial. *There's no gain in containing true emotion.* Tantrums, expressions of rage, wailing, and self-flagellation are excessive—and thankfully they're also rare.

Possibly this fear of expressing feeling, of losing control, makes us feel guarded and safe. The fact is that we are *not* safe. Unexpressed emotions will surface, and they may be more difficult to deal with at a later time. Expressing emotion by crying is taking care of things now, rather than leaving unfinished business we'll have to complete after the fact.

If my mother is dying and I sit at her bedside and shed tears, I have the opportunity to show her how much I love her. I give her, in return, the chance to do her job (to mother me). I can only do this before her life ends. Crying can be relieving and can leave us feeling strengthened. Tears won't wash us away.

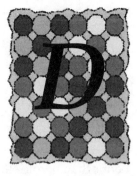

Death

Death is the termination and extinction of life. It's the absence of all signs of living. You'll see that breathing has stopped, and if you feel for a pulse or listen for a heartbeat, neither will be present. At the time of death, the patient will probably lose bladder and bowel control, and the pupils of the eyes will dilate. Electrical measurements of heart and brain activity are absent, although this is not obvious unless the dying person is monitored.

The facial features assume a fixed, waxy expression. In time the skin loses its warmth and becomes cool to the touch. If you are unsure if death has occurred, observe the patient for several minutes, and this will generally confirm the lack of vital life signs. Any competent person may pronounce death, and it's not necessary in every instance to rely upon a physician or nurse.

The law varies in different states, making it important to know the legal requirements in advance.

Dehydration

The human body is composed mostly of water. Water is excreted constantly through the bowel, urine flow, perspiration, and the water vapor present in our breath. Body fluids are replenished by drinking. Normally, when there's excess body water loss, we get thirsty, and then we drink to replace the fluid. Without regular fluid intake, the human body becomes dehydrated. Urine output decreases as the body attempts to hold on to the liquids it has. Other complications may occur that can alter or disrupt blood chemistry, depending on how severe the dehydration has become.

The dehydration that occurs during the dying process isn't accompanied with the same intense thirst a healthy person experiences. Rehydration with intravenous fluids is not useful. Attempting to force fluids into a terminally ill patient may contribute to lung congestion and produce discomfort. Moistening the mouth and lips and making sure the patient's oral hygiene is maintained can provide much comfort. Doing this is usually sufficient, and probably better than heroic efforts to get fluids into the terminally ill patient. If the patient wants to sip fluids, provide them—but never force them on a terminally ill person. Patients sometimes enjoy sucking on flavored ice cubes or popsicles, and offer these freely.

Dementia

Dementia is a chronic, progressive, usually irreversible process. It produces deterioration in memory, language, and behavior. It's not the same as depression, temporary confusion, or delirium. It is *not* a normal part of aging. Thinking and judgment become impaired. Patients may fail to recognize friends or identify objects. Personality changes are usually a part of dementia. Not all dementia is caused by Alzheimer disease, and a neurological evaluation will be essential for proper diagnosis and treatment.

Dementia is a tough problem for families. The patient and family group will require emotional support.

By the time we see patients with dementia in hospice, most of them have had extensive medical investigation. The problems we'll need to handle are those of managing the patient with dementia, not diagnosing the dementia itself. Serious problems include attempts at physical violence, memory loss, and later the loss of physical functions such as swallowing, bowel, and bladder control.

It's common for caregivers to feel angry, frustrated, guilty, and fatigued with trying to manage a patient with dementia. These are *normal* responses to an overwhelming and catastrophic illness. You should seek out a counselor, the hospice social worker, or a chaplain for support. Therapy for the family (as well as the patient) can lessen the stress of dealing with the demented and terminally ill patient.

Denial

Denial is our emotional buffer. It's an unconscious mechanism that cushions us against the painful events in our life. It's a way we can feel safe from threats to our survival. Some people are able to accept slowly the seriousness of their illness. Others can't seem to accept their dying, and will ignore facts as caregivers and physicians present them, or change the subject. Some patients may accept, to some degree, their impending death, but they can't clearly explain how they feel. Denial may also help some patients (and caregivers) get "over the hump" and through the worst part of what's happening.

Because denial allows us to maintain a feeling of safety, don't "break down" or challenge the patient's denial unless it interferes with the patient's ability to function. Often a patient will accept the severity of his or her illness while family members remain in a state of denial. It's best to be truthful, but when a patient doesn't wish to acknowledge information, persisting isn't valuable—it is just a reflection of an unsatisfied need of the person pressing the issue.

Examine *who* needs to recognize what before continuing with an attempt to destroy a patient's denial. I believe there are times when patients are so overwhelmed and gravely ill that delivering bad news is useless.

If we take away denial, we'd better have something better to replace it.

Depression

Depression is a disturbance of mood. Besides producing feelings of sadness and hopelessness, there are physical symptoms that accompany depression, such as loss of appetite and sleep disturbances. Depressed individuals may become irritable and find it difficult to concentrate. When depression is present with no apparent cause, it's called "endogenous depression." Usually depression is a reaction to a specific event or set of events. Depression is common in both patients and families experiencing a terminal illness. Some medications (such as beta-blockers or tranquilizers) can cause depression. If they do, withhold them from the patient. Patients who have been taking a stimulant may experience depression if they stop taking the drug.

When people are depressed, they may feel overwhelmed with despair. They feel that things are not only bad now, but have never been good and *will not improve*. This feeling differs from grief, which is a "normal" reaction to the events surrounding terminal illness.

It's difficult to be around someone who is depressed. Sometimes it seems contagious. We often try to move people out of depression (because we can't stand how we feel when we're around them) by patting them on the shoulder and saying things like, "Come on, cheer up, things will be okay." This frequently drives them further into depression—although unintentionally, of course.

Some patients are annoyed by requests to cheer up. Perhaps they think that the person making the suggestion is taking the situation too lightly. It also may take time for depression to lift, assuming that it does, or it may never lift. Encouraging people to talk about their feelings, and remembering positive past experiences, may help relieve depression.

There are definite chemical changes within the brain that occur during depression. Antidepressant medication can alleviate even deep depression. Some of the medications may take time to work, and may have side effects. Don't discount the idea of using antidepressants to improve the quality of life. Psychotherapy may also relieve some bouts of depression. I sometimes need to remind myself that feelings are not bugs to step on and crush. Feelings need to be felt and honored. Squashing them doesn't work.

Diarrhea

Diarrhea is frequent, watery, or loose stool. It can be accompanied by minor or intense intestinal cramping. If the patient suffers from diarrhea for a long time, it may cause sufficient water loss to produce dehydration and thirst. Administer rehydration and medication to stop diarrhea to improve the patient's comfort. Loss of blood electrolytes such as potassium and sodium are some of the other effects of diarrhea, and you should replace these by a convenient method. It's preferable to replenish fluid and electrolytes orally; try to avoid intravenous treatment. Diarrhea may also occur around a fecal impaction. If there's a change in the patient's bowel habits, the attending physician or nurse should perform a rectal examination.

Dilaudid

Dilaudid is an opiate used frequently to relieve pain. The generic name of this semisynthetic narcotic is hydromorphone. It's available in tablets, suppositories, and solution for intravenous or subcutaneous infusion. It's not available as an oral liquid. Some physicians prefer this medication to morphine, feeling it produces a stronger sensation of euphoria. As with all narcotics, there may be side effects. It's less flexible than morphine, and it is more expensive. If the patient can't tolerate morphine, Dilaudid may be a satisfactory alternative.

Drainage

Drainage is the leaking of fluid from the body. It can occur in many places. Swelling of the arms or legs from obstruction of veins or the lymph channels can cause fluid to seep through the skin. The fluid is usually clear, and the swelling can be reduced by elevating the swollen part.

Catheters, wounds, incisions, and bedsores can also produce seepage. This may be unattractive and foul-smelling. If the opening is infected, antibiotics and frequent cleansing will help. Keep the bedclothes fresh and clean, and the area around the seepage as clean and dry as possible, to reduce the unpleasant odor. Be sure to wash your hands after handling soiled bedclothes or bandages, as this will lessen the chance of spreading infection.

Although drainage may be unsightly and unappealing, it shouldn't be a reason to avoid touching the patient or to refrain from physical contact. Patients need touching and comforting at the end of life.

Dryness

If you apply skin creams to areas of sore or tender skin, you can provide some relief from dryness. There are also several lubricants for the mouth to help patients with dry lips. Refreshing drops for the patient's eyes can be comforting. You can relieve dryness of the nose caused by nasal oxygen by using a mist, or by frequently lubricating the nasal passages. Open-mouth breathing can dry out the mucous membranes. It's important to practice vigorous oral hygiene, and this is something often overlooked (since it was the patient's responsibility prior to the illness).

Dyspnea

Dyspnea refers to difficult breathing or shortness of breath. The patient may have problems breathing if chest movement causes pain. The treatment is pain medication. Patients with lung ailments (for example, tumors and fluid accumulation) may find breathing especially hard work. Removing the fluid may help for awhile, but generally the fluid reaccumulates. Sometimes anxiety can cause "overbreathing" or hyperventilation, and the patient may feel that he or she can't breathe. Severe anemia can also cause dyspnea.

Whatever the cause, dyspnea is a distressing symptom requiring skilled evaluation and specific treatment. There may be circumstances where a specific treatment isn't available. In this case, try to relieve the symptoms with morphine and oxygen. Fortunately, this is usually effective.

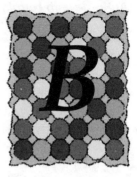

Eating

You should expect loss of appetite with illness, particularly a terminal illness. Dying patients may simply stop eating or restrict their intake to small sips of liquids. There are times when the smell or taste of food is unpleasant to a dying patient. Certain ailments may compress the stomach and restrict the amount of food that the patient can eat. Difficulty swallowing may cause eating to be uncomfortable or painful. When the physician's prognosis is a full recovery, the patient should be encouraged to eat. With a dying patient, food can be offered, but you shouldn't force it. Forced feeding can be a burden and is emotionally distressing. There are many other ways to show love and concern.

The purpose of food at this time is enjoyment *not* nutrition.

Embarrassment

The period of dying can be stressful for everyone. We're likely to see examples of the best and the worst in the people involved. As stress-filled as it is, the end of life can represent a tremendous opportunity for growth, both for the dying person and for the caregivers. Caregivers may have thoughts and feelings that they are hesitant to express because they feel embarrassed. Try to work through this inhibition and say what you feel. Feel free to express what's on your mind. Waiting until later, until you think it's more appropriate, or until you've got it worked out exactly how you'll say it, might lead to you missing a chance at powerful communication.

There is no better time than the present to express what's in your heart. There may not be a time later to do so.

Euthanasia

Euthanasia is the act of killing a person painlessly because doing so seems "merciful." It's commonly called "mercy killing." Euthanasia is a way to kill the pain by killing the one who suffers. You must ask yourself: *Whose pain are we killing? Ours or the person who is dying?* With suicide, the choice is the victim's—and he is also the perpetrator. In euthanasia (as in murder) a second person becomes responsible for taking another's life.

Most physicians, while empathetic with the feelings behind it, are uncomfortable with laws that empower them to take away life. This is contrary to the physician's Hippocratic oath to do no harm.

There are instances where euthanasia may seem to be the only acceptable alternative to prolonged and agonizing suffering. Advocates of both sides of the issue provide convincing arguments for their positions.

Advocates of euthanasia justify their belief in "mercy killing" by citing many examples of patients who die in horrible unrelieved pain. When I've examined these reports, I usually find a few common facts about them:

1. They are reported by people who have been personally and emotionally involved, and not all the facts have been presented.
2. Good medical evaluation and therapy wasn't provided prior to choosing euthanasia.
3. The patients didn't have access to hospice or weren't on a hospice program.
4. The patient was in a setting where the primary focus wasn't on providing good pain management and palliative care.

There do exist patients for whom pain doesn't respond to treatment. And if we continue increasing the dosage of narcotics for pain control, the patient can succumb to an overdose. Better that this happen, where the primary motivation is helping (regardless of side effects), than euthanasia—where the goal is termination. Physicians are trained to heal and to save life. It doesn't require much training or skill to kill.

Even with the strictest laws, there's always the chance that euthanasia will become the most expedient way to resolve society's issues. The choice to end a life involves a very complex personal decision, and it shouldn't be resolved in the political arena. There is something uncivilized about taking life. Although I can sometimes intellectually rationalize the act (as in "putting a pet to sleep"), the feelings about committing the act of terminating human life aren't so easy to dispel. While I'm not comparing humans to pets, the feelings about ending a life of someone or something we love are similar. I'd hate to see the day when professionals become so emotionally removed that euthanasia becomes an easily accepted and rationalized act. Perhaps we had a taste of this in Nazi Germany.

Most hospice professionals believe that if we provide good enough care for the terminally ill, and relieve physical, emotional, and spiritual pain, euthanasia shouldn't be an option. Therefore, the issue is the *quality of the patient's care*, not the reasons for or against taking life. Provide satisfactory care and euthanasia shouldn't become an attractive idea.

I made a home visit to a man who had severe, unrelenting pain in an area above his bladder. This required irrigation three or four times a day, and he screamed each time the nurse worked on the area. When I saw him he asked me to kill him. He couldn't live with the pain—and with the thought that it would continue until he died. I asked him just what he thought it would take to make him change his mind about wanting to die. He said he could live only if he was rid of this horrible pain.

I changed his pain medication and adjusted the treatment schedule so that by the next day he was comfortable and smiling—and able to tolerate the treatments. He had been on several other drugs and they had not relieved his pain. The proper changes allowed him to be comfortable.

Good hospice care with aggressive pain and symptom control can go a long way to shortening the list of candidates for euthanasia.

I would like to say a few words about suicide and physician-assisted suicide. Several states have introduced initiatives to legalize physician-assisted suicide. They are doing this because many are discontented with the way people are allowed to die, or in some cased, forced to die. I believe that hospice is an alternative to euthanasia.

In the United States hospice care has been available to the terminally ill through the Medicare program. Access to this benefit has been limited partly because of the reluctance of physicians to accept dying and discuss hospice in a forthright manner as an *opportunity* for a patient. Patients usually need a physician's referral to get into a hospice program. Hospice isn't the answer for everybody with a terminal illness, and for those who begin a hospice program, there is no guarantee that all the pain and symptoms will be controlled. There are times when we're not completely successful even when we do all that we can possibly do.

Sometimes to relieve suffering we need to administer large doses of narcotics—doses sufficient to result in death. If the patient dies, the doctor's intention wasn't to kill, but to relieve pain. This is sometimes called "the double-edged sword." I'm sure that there are times when a physician's intentions might be ambiguous. In most cases, the doctor wants what the patient wants—a comfortable and peaceful death. Some patients may ask for help to die, or they might ask for information regarding a means to kill themselves.

While I don't support the idea of suicide as a way out or pain, I respect that a person ought to have a choice, if possible, in the way their life ends. Even if the person doesn't end up choosing suicide, the knowledge that they have that option and the means to execute it can be relieving. The person knows that he or she still has some control over the end of life, and the means to terminate life if it becomes intolerable. I think this philosophy is in keeping with our mission as caregivers to relieve emotional pain (worry and fear) and enhance the quality of life.

The end of life can be a period of growth, both emotionally and spiritually. Hospice offers choice: a chance for closure, for completion of life tasks, for live review, and for celebration of our value as worthwhile persons. Euthanasia and assisted suicide eliminate this opportunity.

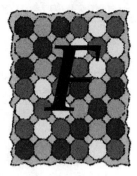

Family

The family is the basic unit with which the hospice is involved. Trained hospice professionals understand that each family is a complex system with established interactions, behaviors, and responses. The period of dying puts immense stress on the family, and on each individual involved. The family, as noted in the preface, is like a delicately balanced mobile—when one member of the family changes, all members are affected. Relationships during this time of duress may become strained (or strengthened). Strain may precipitate disagreements.

Also, family members whose contact with those close to the patient has been superficial might arrive on the scene with lots of "advice" on how to handle things. They may feel guilty for not having participated in the family core, and attempt to "take over." They might suggest new treatments or consultations or make unwanted comments on how to improve the carefully established hospice structure. These people usually mean well, but they may need to be advised that the way the patient is being cared for in the best way, and that the current method will continue despite their suggestions.

It's difficult to advise family members living far away from a dying patient when is the best time to visit. It's rarely possible to predict the time of death so all family members interested can be present. Each person must decide upon the time to come. The earlier the better, since it is important to avoid missing the opportunity for personal closure with a loved one. Some people can arrange to spend weeks or months in the home of a dying person. Others may not be able to alter their lives much, and may need to say their good-byes early.

Fatigue

The long and intense involvement in caring for the dying can cause emotional and physical fatigue. Constant worry and lack of rest from providing around-the-clock medications can exact a heavy toll on a caregiver. If it's affordable, hiring a helper can give caregivers a chance to rest.

Respite care for a short time in a skilled nursing facility will lighten the load. Don't be afraid to ask for assistance—it's not a reflection of any weakness or lack of dedication on your part. Ask the hospice social worker, nurse, friends, and hospice volunteers to help you.

Sometimes fatigue becomes overwhelming, and one simply can't manage the patient at home. It isn't a failure if one has to move the patient out of the home and into professional hands. The patient may benefit from the skilled care, and rested caregivers should be able to spend quality time wjith the patient at the end.

Remember, as overwhelming and endless as it seems, there will be an end.

Fear

While there are imaginary fears, there are also real fears. Patients may equate cancer with an agonizing death, or may have seen someone die in pain. Encouraging patients to talk about their fears is a good practice. It's best to address the fear head on and work for a solution to it than avoid it—and possibly have it grow larger and more troublesome.

Listen with that "third ear" that lets us hear the real message behind the words. Patients (and caregivers) don't often say, "I'm scared" or "I'm so frightened." They're more likely to act out, to hide, or to ask such things as: "How long is this going to go on?" or say "I don't know what I'm going to do," or just look frightened.

I once spoke with a woman dying of lung cancer. Her husband had suffocated because of lung cancer, and she was terrified at suffering a similar fate. He had died a few years earlier and had not had the benefit of hospice. This woman's life ended comfortably and peacefully. It was important that I discussed her fear with her, and even more so that I correctly reassured her that she wouldn't suffer as her husband had.

Fluids

At the end of life, patients will drink less. Some may stop eating and drinking or be content with a few sips. Dehydration, a serious concern in patients expected to recover, isn't a concern in the dying. *Overhydration* is far worse and may cause discomfort, swelling, and lung congestion. Forcing fluids—particularly in patients who have trouble swallowing—can cause choking. Offer fluids, keep the patient's mouth moist, but abandon the idea of "making" the patient drink. It's often enough to have the patient suck on ice cubes, flavored ice, or popsicles. Good oral hygiene is a must.

Intravenous fluids are a mainstay in medical treatment. Fluids are given to replace losses, such as from vomiting or diarrhea, and they can make up defects in people who've been deprived of water. Elderly persons in skilled nursing facilities may be tied down or restricted by side rails from reaching for water to drink. Adding water intravenously to weak and dehydrated patients can make "instant people." This isn't the case in dying patients. Intravenous lines are also used to administer vitamins, antibiotics, and nutrients to patients unable to eat or swallow. In most cases, vitamins, nutrients, and antibiotics are useless to the dying.

Some people seem to think that withholding food and fluids at the end of life is cruel or negligent. If this were the same as backing off from meaningful treatment and it caused discomfort, it would be wrong. In the case of the dying, it's sufficient to maintain good mouth care. If the patient doesn't want to eat, respect the patient's wish.

In the intensive care setting where we expect patients to recover, and everybody is actively trying to keep a person alive, we say, "Don't just stand there, *do something*." In a hospice setting, where frustration comes from helplessness and the hard realization that there isn't a lot to do, we say, "Don't just do something, *be there*."

I want to emphasize that patients do not become dehydrated in the conventional sense, and it's wrong to believe (and poor hospice care to insist) that all patients who are not drinking require immediate intravenous hydration.

Forgiveness

The primary task in the period of bereavement is forgiveness. It may appear difficult to do. Only through forgiveness can survivors emerge from grief and begin to function again. The process begins with forgiving an unfair world where bad things happen to good people. Try to forgive a medical establishment that is sometimes fragmented, doesn't have all the answers, and sometimes doesn't seem to care. We can try to forgive those who have not been as attentive and supportive as we wish they had. We can try to forgive the person who died and abandoned us. In the case of a religious person, the individual can try to come to terms with a God who let the death of a loved one happen.

Most important of all, we can forgive ourselves for not living up to our own expectations.

Remember: *We are only human.*

Fractures

Bone strength can decrease when patients are bed-bound and inactive. Cancer that invades bone can cause areas of weakness so that simple twisting or turning may fracture a bone. Fractures occur not only in long bones of the arms and legs, but also occur in the spinal vertebrae and the ribs. Fractures hurt when moved and may put pressure on nearby nerves, causing weakness or pain.

Radiation therapy is effective in areas where cancer has spread to the bone, but the patient's condition may not allow trips to the hospital for radiation. Fractures that would ordinarily be pinned and stabilized may not be treatable in the usual manner, because the patient is too ill.

Carefully evaluate the balance between the quality of remaining life and the risks involved in surgical procedure. One can stabilize fractures without surgery and provide comfort at the end of life without adding the trauma of invasive procedures.

Fractures can happen in any bone in the body, particularly in older patients whose bones and weak or affected by disease. Treatment usually requires that one immobilize the fractured bone until it knits back together. This can take as long as six or eight weeks, depending on the bone and the patient's health. We can pin hip fractures, but the patient won't be able to bear weight on that leg right away. A total hip replacement might be appropriate for a person expected to recover and walk soon after surgery.

Since both these surgeries (pinning and replacement) require a general anesthetic and are stressful to the body, so rarely—if ever—are these correct treatments for a terminally ill patient. Casts can stabilize certain fractures while they heal (and new types of casts are much lighter than the old plaster type). If the patient is days or weeks from death, it may be kinder simply to immobilize the fractured area, or splint the arm or leg that's broken and leave it at that.

Radiation therapy can treat spinal fractures where there's a chance the spinal cord might compress and cause paralysis below the fracture. First, confirm the fracture by X-ray, and then start the radiation treatment. Here, again, the risk-to-benefit ratio comes into play. The results of X-ray treatment aren't immediate, and you must take into account the time and energy spent transporting the patient (as well as the patient's discomfort while being moved).

Some physicians prefer to try steroid therapy (oral cortisone) first, thinking that if the patient doesn't respond to steroids, radiation isn't likely to help either.

The old adage—*The punishment should fit the crime*—is still true.

Remember that many medical decisions are educated guesses based on the doctor's experience and modified by the patient's wishes and also by the patient's family. When we look back at our decisions, not every one will be 100 percent correct. We need to remember that under the circumstances, we used our best judgment and did the best that we could do.

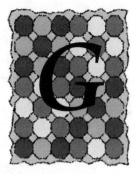

Gas

When gas accumulates in the stomach or the rest of the bowel, it produces a feeling of pressure, fullness, bloating, or distension. Releasing the gas reduces the stretching of the gut and should provide relief. Pressure caused by a tumor or fluid in the abdomen can cause a similar feeling, often mistaken for gas, but not as easily relieved. Sometimes you can drain fluid, but it's likely to recur. The physician can place a tube in the intestinal tract through the nose or rectum, but remember to weigh the discomfort of the tube against the discomfort of the gas.

Antispasmodic drugs may help the cramping that accompanies gas. In some situations, narcotics can worsen intestinal cramping, and this will make it harder to provide relief. The essential thing to do is weigh the potential complications of providing relief against the discomfort caused by the gas. If the technique used to relieve the gas will hurt more than the gas, how does it improve the quality of the patient's life?

Grief

Grief is the sorrow that we experience when we lose something or someone dear to us. Experiencing grief is normal. You should become concerned when a caregiver or loved one fails to grieve— or experiences prolonged or pathologically deep grief. You might begin feeling grief before a loved one dies. This is anticipatory grief. It's doesn't make the loss any easier to accept, but it may help you work through some of the deep emotions. Although most people recover from grief, the feelings that come with it can be overwhelming.

Remember: *Active grieving = time = healing.*

Consider getting professional assistance (counseling) and participating in a group with others who've experienced the death of a loved one. Don't contain your grief—share your feelings of loss with others close to you. It will help you and the person with whom you speak. It's a terrible myth that the way to experience loss is to suffer in quiet and try to cap off the boiling emotions that come with profound loss.

There is no grief which time does not lessen and soften.

— Cicero, *Epistolae*, IV.v.

Grunting

Patients in a stupor (or semicomatose) may make grunting, groaning, or moaning sounds. These don't always mean the patient is suffering from pain or distress. When you're moving, lifting, or turning a patient, and this causes a facial grimace or a groan, that probably means the action is painful for the patient.

Patients often have trouble swallowing in the late stages of dying, but they can usually absorb liquid painkillers. You can administer liquid morphine, and soluble morphine tablets placed inside the patient's cheek or under the tongue should help. Be sure to check to see what's causing the pain before rushing to use painkillers.

Things as simple as an obstructed urinary catheter or pressure on a sensitive area such as a fractured rib are easy to correct, and doing so eliminates the need to add another drug to the patient's system.

Guilt

Guilt frequently is a worthless and destructive emotion—unless it acts as a motivation to change undesirable behavior and point us in another more positive direction. Caregivers commonly feel guilty for lots of things. They may think that they didn't recognize the signs of illness quickly enough, they fear that they haven't been persistent enough about urging treatment, they may think that they didn't do enough to help or that they've made mistakes with medication, they become short-tempered, angry, frustrated, and on and on.

We are our own harshest judge—and often a ruthless jury.

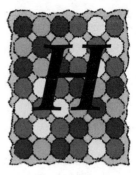

Hair

The most common problem with hair is that it falls out. Chemotherapy or radiation therapy have the unfortunate side effect of making most patients lose their hair. Also, when the hair follicles recover and the hair grows back, it can be darker, grey, straighter, coarser, and so on. Many people derive pride from their appearance, so keep in mind how stressful it can be to wake up and find most of your hair on the pillow.

Some surgical procedures require that the patient's head get shaved, although this generally doesn't change the condition of the hair when it grows back.

If the patient wants a wig or cap to cover the scalp, provide one.

Hallucination

Hallucinating is the experience of seeing or hearing something that doesn't exist. Hallucinations are a product of the mind when it's under physical, chemical, or emotional stress. Visual and auditory hallucinations are common in dying patients. They may be the result of complicated metabolic processes, or they may be due to the interactions of drugs in the patient's system. Dying patients are sensitive, and drugs they might have tolerated when they were healthy may create hallucinations.

Cardiac medication, such as digoxin (Lanoxin), which is usually safe, may cause problems in the dying. Reevaluate all nonessential and nonpalliative medications. Discontinue administering any drugs not required to maintain the patient's comfort. However, do not stop administering drugs without consulting the hospice doctor or nurse first. Sometimes patients may require medication if they become disturbed by their hallucinations.

As always, calm and gentle reassurance is helpful.

Hearing

Thirty years ago, when I was a resident physician in internal medicine at the Los Angeles Country General Hospital, I read a book about the care of the aged, the dying, and the dead. I remember the part that described how we place the dying—with their diminished sight—in a darkened room, and we whisper around those with decreased ability to hear.

In our efforts to maintain an appropriately somber and respectful environment, we whisper the word "cancer" and tiptoe about, creating a morguelike atmosphere before it's time to do so. Hearing may diminish at the end of life. Speak loudly enough for the dying person to hear, and make an effort to create a cheerful, pleasant, and comfortable environment.

The dying patient, as is true for all patients, probably does not wish to feel as if he or she is all alone. Speak up. The patient wants to hear what you have to say.

Hope

Hope is a combination of our desire for something and our expectation that the desire will be fulfilled. Dying patients usually retain a glimmer of hope, but the nature of their hope may change. Patients who once thought of living a long time simply hope for living a little longer. When that's impossible, they hope for comfort, the avoidance of pain, and for closeness with others.

To some extent, hope is wishful thinking. It's dreaming that something outside of ourselves will appear and rescue us, tell us that this isn't really happening, and save us from the tragedy that we're experiencing. In a sense, hope is a delusion. Dying will not disappear, and we will each have to do it by ourselves. Friends and loved ones can help along the path, but they cannot, finally, die for you.

We hope we can have a comfortable and meaningful closure. This should be the mutual goal of patients and family. Sometimes patients have secret wishes about which they feel shy or embarrassed. Ask the patient about these; if they are still within the realm of possibility, try to make them come true.

> While there's life, there's hope.
>
> —Cicero, *Ad Atticum*, IX.x.

Hospice

People usually think of hospice as a facility—a place that provides supportive care for the dying. Actually, hospice is a philosophy of providing pain and symptom control, or "palliative care," to terminally ill patients. We usually provide hospice in the home. We can also provide hospice care in the hospital or in a special hospice building or skilled nursing facility.

I would like to share with you another view of hospice. Hospice is more than a place that serves the dying and it is more than the philosophy and the art and the science of palliation at the end of life. Hospice is really an embodiment of all of us who do this work of caring for the dying. It is our personification. If I were a hospice and I could talk, this is what I'd say:

> I welcome you who have illness beyond cure and who are dying. Even if you don't accept your dying or don't choose to know. I welcome you. I sincerely believe that when cure is no longer possible, you still need to be cared for and cared about. I do that. . . . I care. I relieve your pain and suffering as best I can. I treat your physical pain—you deserve to be comfortable and not waste the time at the end of your life hurting. Then I can treat your emotional pain, your sadness, and your fears about dying and I can treat your spiritual pain and attend to your spiritual needs because you have a human spirit that needs to be nurtured now—more than ever—and should not be ignored. I am hospice. I am here to celebrate you as a person who is important and worthwhile simply

because you are. I'm here to hold you, to comfort you, and to love you at the end of your life.

Michael Appleton, 1993

Humor

Dying isn't funny, yet there are some humorous things that happen in the transition from life to death. Sometimes it's hard for us to keep a straight face. It's not necessary to remain forever somber and serious. While it's disrespectful to laugh at the plight of a person who is dying, laughing *with* them and sharing humorous things can be a valuable and wonderful way of bonding. I'm talking about laughter as a relieving—even palliative—force. The power of shared humor can provide some relief for both people.

Sometimes a mispronunciation such as calling a pacemaker a peacemaker can bring on a chuckle. On one of my home visits a patient offered me a bowl of candy. This was the third visit in a row where people pushed candy on me. Did I look as if I had a chocolate bar deficiency? When I accepted the third offering of the morning, the patient told me that one of the hospice nurses said that I loved candy. We all had a laugh about how puzzled I'd been, and how I'd had such a hard time figuring out who spilled the beans on my habit.

Another time I was leaning over a bed, examining a very drowsy old woman. She opened her eyes and asked: "So who's this?" I couldn't just say, "I'm the doctor," so I whispered into her ear, "I'm the handsome prince charming coming to pick you up for the Saturday night dance." She smiled and said, "You wouldn't be tryin' to fool an old lady, would you?"

Many things happen in the course of terminal illness. Dying brings out the best and the worst in people. One of the best things is the ability to play and enjoy a bit of humor—it's part of our essence, part of our *humanness*, and something we all can share.

Hydration

See fluids, dehydration.

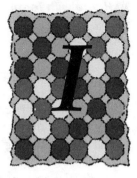

Impaction

Fecal impaction is the presence of hard stool that blocks the bowel and is difficult to pass. It's common in terminal illness because inactivity slows the bowel, and changes in diet (such as drinking less fluids) make the fecal matter dry and hard. Many medications—particularly opiates—make the smooth muscles of the bowel move less, and this retards the normal process of pushing the bolus (digested food mass) through the bowel.

You should probably anticipate that the patient will suffer from constipation and impaction. Impaction causes discomfort, and the removing feces manually can be painful. Start using laxatives and stool softeners early. The patient may also need frequent rectal examinations to preempt complications farther down the road.

Incisions

Surgical incisions may not heal well, or they can reopen in terminally ill patients whose metabolic processes aren't functioning well. Restitching is often impractical. Taping the wound together with butterfly "stitches" should suffice. There might be multiple incisions that haven't healed, and they may all drain quite a bit.

You should keep the surrounding areas as clean as possible, and take care of the skin around the incision—it's likely to get inflamed. This might be the best you can do. If an enterostomal therapist (a person specializing in the care of incisions and openings in the body) is available, seek that person's advice on how to treat your particular patient's problems.

Incontinence

If the patient loses control of bowel or bladder, change the patient's diapers frequently to reduce odor and prevent the bed-clothes from getting soiled. If the patient's skin is constantly wet with urine, it may break down and become irritated and infected. In that case a urinary catheter might be a necessary trade-off. Try your best to keep the area dry before resorting to a catheter.

It's also important to remember that the patient can be embarrassed by the need to wear diapers and to be cleaned. Reassure them that the problem isn't their fault and doesn't reflect badly on them.

Infection

As people approach the end of life, they are less able to fight infection. The patient's muscles grow weaker, and they're less able to cough, increasing the chances of pneumonia. Oral infections with monilia (candida) are common. Monilial infection can also occur in moist body areas such as the groin, armpits, and under the breasts. Expect to see infections of the urinary tract if the patient has a urinary catheter. Skin infections and infected bedsores may occur, too.

Base the decision to treat or not to treat infections upon the anticipated response of the infection to antibiotics. If the outcome will be to increase comfort and the quality of life, then it's desirable to treat the infection. If all it's likely to do is prolong dying, then avoid adding another drug to the patient's treatment. With people who are expected to recover, aggressive antibiotic therapy can be life-saving. For the terminally ill patient, the same therapy may be useless and—at best—prolong the dying process.

Each choice to treat or to withhold therapy must be an individual decision. The decision should be made jointly by the family, the patient, and the physician.

Intravenous Fluids

Intravenous fluids are used to replace lost body fluid and to provide hydration when the patient isn't taking in enough liquid by mouth. They're also used as a vehicle for administering many medications. If we're deprived of water, we become thirsty. Usually we're able to drink enough to replenish lost body fluids. Dehydration at the end of life is usually symptomless and doesn't require rehydration. Especially *not* with intravenous fluids. Additional fluids can cause the patient's weakened system to overload and will complicate their illness.

Just because intravenous fluids have been started isn't a good reason to continue them. There's no obligation to keep doing it once it's obvious that there's no benefit. Intravenous infusions with morphine, though, are effective for pain control when the patient can't take medicine by mouth. Subcutaneous (under-the-skin) infusions are easier to manage and are just as effective. Terminal illness can be treated without resorting to intravenous fluids, so avoid them.

Caregivers sometimes become anxious because, "Grandma isn't eating or drinking and may dehydrate." Actually, more problems occur if you overhydrate a patient. Providing I.V. fluids to dying patients may—at best—prolong the dying process. Fluids can cause complications by adversely altering the body chemistry of the patient and can cause lung congestion and difficulty breathing at the end.

Remember: *Keeping patients dry keeps them comfortable.*

Isolation

Dying patients fear abandonment and frequently feel alone and isolated. This fear is aggravated by being shut off in a sterile hospital room and separated from the sight and sound of life. Even though dying is a process that no one can do for us, we shouldn't have to be alone or feel lonely at the time of death. Familiar surroundings and a sense of home—with friends and family nearby—can make the journey easier.

Our human need for company isn't lessened by the nearness of death. Sit with a dying loved one and share their remaining days. It'll be a time rich with personal growth for both you and the terminally ill person.

Itching

Pruritus is the medical term for itching. Itching varies from mild to severe. There are many causes of itching, including allergy, infection, and jaundice. Allergic reactions to medications such as sulfa drugs or penicillin sometimes produce itching hives. Moist areas of the body where the skin has gotten raw may itch, too. Avoid using skin medications that contain lots of oil. You might have to use topical cortisone or antihistamines and anesthetic lotions to provide relief from maddening itching.

Severe itching may require systemic steroids (cortisone) and antihistamines such as benadryl, hydroxyzine (Atarax), or Temaril. The long-term side effects of systemic cortisone use aren't an issue here, but maximum relief from maddening itching is. Do whatever you can to relieve itching.

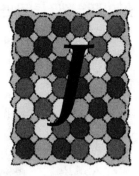

Jargon

Jargon is the specialized language of a group. Golfers have a special lingo when they talk about Eagles and Birdies. Computer lingo uses Kbytes, megs, pixels, icons, and so on. Medical jargon is the same way. It's the language that medical professionals use to talk about their work. Jargon saves time and a lot of explanation. We assume that the in-crowd understands when we throw around terms such as "azotemia" and "conduction defects." Jargon makes me appear wise as I toss it off while talking to other physicians.

We physicians sometimes use jargon to make ourselves sound impressive and knowledgeable. It identifies us as being "in the group." We're in the know, we speak the same language. It's also used as shorthand for commonly repeated terms or procedures.

The problem is that while it seems to bring the "group" closer together, it can distance and alienate others. They feel left out. Think about how you feel at a dinner table where everyone else speaks a language you do not understand. It's a pretty cold sensation.

Jargon can be used to hide feelings. The more uncomfortable I become, the easier it is to "jargonize" things. I appear all knowing, and I distance myself from my discomfort. This is the same as calling death "passing on." It serves the same purpose but in a different manner.

It's not always easy to be straightforward and use plain down-home language. But speaking simply in an emotionally charged situation is essential if what I want is to *communicate* and bring me and my patients closer together.

Beware of jargon—ask for explanations that make sense. If you don't understand something, it's not a bad thing to ask to have it explained to you.

Some common buzzwords and jargon follow, with simple definitions. This list isn't complete, but it's a start. It isn't intended as a dictionary, just a list of a few of the most common terms you'll see and hear.

ABG	arterial blood gas.
AC	before meals (1/2 h AC means 1/2 hour before meals).
Acyclovir	Zovirax, a medication for herpes, shingles.
ASAP	as soon as possible.
AZT	Zidovudine, the primary drug used to inhibit the AIDS, or HIV virus.
BID	twice a day, usually every 12 hours.
CATH	catheter, a tube placed into the bladder for drainage of urine.
cc	same as cubic centimeter, same as ml, or milliliter. Five cc or 5 ml equals 1 teaspoon, 0.5 cc equals 1/2 cc or 1/2 ml, 30 cc equals 1 ounce, 1000 cc equals 1 liter, or about 1 quart.
CMV	cytomeglovirus, an infection in AIDS patients that causes blindness.
CPR	cardiopulmonary resuscitation; a method of closed-chest massage and coordinated breathing assistance used to revive a person who has had a cardiac arrest. *A cardiac arrest is usually the manner of death for a terminally ill patient for whom no recovery is espected. To call paramedics or to perform CPR in such a case is not only useless, but it can also add suffering and agony at the moment of death.*
DC	discontinue, stop.
DHPG	Gancyclovir, a drug used to treat CMV.
DISP#	dispense number, how many (written on a prescription).
DNR	do not resuscitate. This is standard for "no heroic measures." This means no CPR.
ETOH	alcohol.
GTT	drops.

HIV	human immunodeficiency virus, the cause of AIDS.
HS	at bedtime, or hour of sleep.
i, ii, iii, iv, v, vi	same as 1, 2, 3, 4, 5, 6.
IM	intramuscular, an injection into muscle tissue.
IV	intravenous, an injection or infusion by vein.
LPM	liters per minute, used to rate the flow of oxygen.
MAI	a type of tuberculosis common in AIDS.
MEDS	medications.
METS	same as metastases, or the spread of cancer to other areas of the body.
OID	once a day, same as QD.
PCP	pneumocystis, Carinii pneumonia, a common respiratory infection in AIDS patients.
PO	per orum, or oral administration.
PR	per rectum, or rectal administration
PRN	as needed for, PRN pain equals as needed for pain.
Q	every (period). So Q40 equals every 4 hours.
QID	four times a day, usually every 6 hours.
Shot	injection.
SIG	directions on how to take a medication (on prescription).
SQ	subcutaneous, or under the skin.
STAT	now, immediate.
TB	tuberculosis.
TB drugs	INH, Rifampin, Ethionamide, used in treating tuberculosis.
TID	three times a day, usually every 8 hours.
TMP	sulfa (Septra, Bactrim), an antibacterial drug to treat urinary infections, also used to treat PCP.
Vital signs	refers to blood pressure, pulse, and respiration— all the signs of life cease at the time of death (but not always together).

Jaundice

Bile is excreted from the liver, stored in the gallbladder, and passed through the bile ducts into the intestine where it emulsifies (helping to digest) fat. When the patient's liver function is impaired, or when there's an obstruction to the bile ducts, bilrubin accumulates in the blood. Eventually, this substance is carried throughout the bloodstream to all the tissues of the body, and it causes a yellow stain, or *jaundice*. We see the discoloration in the whites of the eyes, and in the patient's skin.

Jaundice is common with malignancies that obstruct the bile ducts in the pancreas. While it doesn't have any dangerous symptoms, severe jaundice can cause intense itching. Because the bile content of the blood is high (from its inability to pass into the intestinal tract), the stool is light and clay colored, while the urine looks like dark tea.

Joints

A prolonged stay in bed can cause stiff joints. If the patient is always lying in one position and rarely moving, the long skeletal muscles can contract. In extended bed-ridden illness, such as a lengthy coma, even the connective tissue at the joints can shorten, creating intense pain when the patient tries to move. To prevent this, gently move the patient's limbs several times a day.

You might also want to apply heating pads prior to moving the joint, which should help loosen it. Administer additional pain medication, or move the patient after a regular dose to help lessen the discomfort.

Physical therapy (as we know it for regular injuries) has a different place with the terminally ill patient. The physical therapist's role in hospice is to keep the patient comfortable and teach caregivers the best ways to move the patient. Exercising the patient (and possibly causing pain) for any other reason is undesirable, since the individual is not expected to recover. Causing suffering while trying to increase mobility is pointless. Consultation with a physical therapist is usually a good idea.

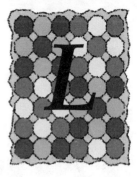

Lips

Mouth breathing and dehydration can cause lips to dry and crack. Lubrication and moistening helps. Herpes (cold sores) that appear as painful blisters, and later as a crust, can be treated with acyclovir cream (Zovirax). Cracking and redness at the edges of the mouth may be due to vitamin B depletion, and sometimes it will respond to supplemental vitamins.

Oral monilia (candida or thrush) can also cause soreness and redness of the mouth and produce an irritation at the edges of the mouth, and this is what I see the most. This usually responds to rinses, gargles, and lozenges that contain an antifungal agent such as Mycostatin.

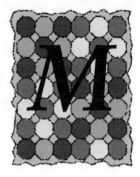

Massage

Touching and massage can be an important part of the healing process. Touching seems particularly important at the extremes of life: infancy and at the end of life. Gentle massage of muscles can be relieving and is a valuable way of communicating. Meaningful human contact is usually a pleasurable experience for patients.

Take care, however, to avoid brisk rubbing, and if the patient's skin becomes irritated, or if the patient feels discomfort, discontinue the massage.

Medications

Medications that a patient needed before may become unnecessary during the final weeks or days of terminal illness. Some drugs have a narrow margin of safety. This means that there's only a small difference between a safe dose and a toxic dose. While a particular dose might be okay in a normal patient, the same dosage might be dangerous to a dying patient.

In the case of older patients and dying patients who have lost weight, you may have to reduce the dosages of (or in some cases stop administering) certain drugs. Review all medications frequently with a professional such as a the patient's physician or the hospice nurse. Discontinue drugs that aren't essential to the patient's well-being.

Remember: *Always check with the doctor before changing a patient's drug schedule, or have the hospice nurse talk to the doctor about it.*

Drugs to alleviate high blood pressure can lower the patient's blood pressure to a dangerous level. Drugs that drop blood sugar in diabetics may cause hypoglycemia and severe side effects in patients with reduced food intake and weight loss. A patient who isn't eating and isn't taking in adequate fluid should probably stop diuretics and potassium supplements.

A good piece of advice when it comes to giving medicine to a terminally ill patient is: *When in doubt, leave it out.*

One exception to the general rule about using smaller doses is the use of pain medication such as morphine. We expect that as a disease that causes pain progresses, so will the amount of morphine required to control the pain. Increased pain doesn't always indicate worsening of the disease, but it does require a prompt increase in pain medication. Sometimes patients will require (and tolerate) huge doses of morphine. There shouldn't be an "upper limit" to the dosage. Increase the dose progressively to match the need for pain control.

Use tranquilizers, antidepressants, and sleeping medications carefully. Don't use these to treat a caregiver who's having difficulty coping with a patient's anxiety, depression, or insomnia. Get skilled professional advice to help that problem.

The goal is to keep the patient comfortable and functional. There are times, however, when patients are so unmanageable that heavy sedation is an acceptable option.

If a patient finds it hard to swallow (as can be the case) you can administer liquid medication by mouth or use rectal suppositories. You can relieve the patient's pain with sublingual (under the tongue) morphine that's absorbed through the membranes of the patient's mouth. Special adhesive patches containing opiates (such as transdermal Fentanyl or Duragesic) provide a continuous level of the drug as it is absorbed through the patient's skin.

Subcutaneous infusion (infusing the medication in fluid under the skin) has generally replaced the need for an intravenous route. The old-fashioned "shot" with a hypodermic needle hurts.

Monilia

See thrush, candida, burning mouth.

Morphine

Morphine is a narcotic. It closely resembles the body's own natural pain-relieving opiates, the endorphins. Sometimes we call morphine God's medicine, because of its miraculous ability to relieve pain. Morphine has gotten a lot of bad press. Concerns about addiction and respiratory depression are just some of the "problems" this inexpensive and very effective drug is supposed to have.

Morphine is addictive, but fear of addiction is misplaced when you're treating the dying patient. Don't withhold morphine because you're afraid the patient may become addicted. Start it early and gradually increase the dosage to maintain effective pain relief. Don't reserve it for "the end."

There are side effects to any medication, and morphine certainly isn't an exception. Drowsiness, confusion, and nausea are not allergic reactions. They're side effects that generally diminish or disappear with continued use. Morphine always causes constipation, so treat it in advance with a vigorous bowel program.

Overdosing and abuse of morphine is rare. Physicians who dwell on these issues usually are inexperienced using opiates to control the pain of dying patients. A large part of the medical profession continues to uncritically accept these myths about morphine—and they do so the detriment of the terminally ill patient. Many people who have been unable to rest because of pain seem to sleep too much after receiving morphine. They sleep because they can rest without discomfort.

Mouth

Mouth care (oral hygiene) is an important part of tending to the terminally ill patient. Mouth breathing can dry out the mucous membranes, and mucous can become thick and difficult to remove. Oxygen also dries out the mucous membranes. The patient's gums may shrink and dentures won't fit correctly.

Canker sores are common. Food debris may accumulate in the patient's mouth and between the teeth. Clean the patient's teeth frequently, and lubricate and moisten the patient's mouth if it gets dry. You must treat mouth infections and keep the patient's mouth as clean as possible. Also remember that some people are embarrassed to be seen without their dentures.

Movement

Weakness and pain may make it hard for the patient to move. With prolonged disuse, the muscles in the arms and legs shorten, and muscular contractions happen that further limit how much they can be moved. Be gentle when you try to move the patient's extremities, but gradually try to increase the limb's mobility. Massage and gentle stretching can help as long as it's not painful.

When it hurts for the patient to move a limb, the patient moves the limb less—making it even stiffer—increasing the muscle atrophy and weakness, making it more painful...and so on.

Physical therapy would be appropriate here only as a method of making it less painful for the patient to move a limb, not as treatment designed to get the patient "back to normal."

Music

Recently, while visiting the home of a patient of mine who was dying of AIDS, I spoke with a woman who was laying on the bed with the patient. She was talking to him and caressing him. Pachelbel's Canon in D was playing on the stereo. This lovely piece reminded me how important music can be in the home where a person is dying. It could be the patient's favorite music or any soft and soothing melody that sets a peaceful tone and allows the caregivers and the patient to relax and feel less burdened.

The music needn't be somber or funereal—nor do rap or a marching band seem quite right. The best choice would be music that celebrates life and brings comfort to the listener.

In silence there can be quiet pain. Music can lift the spirit and massage the soul.

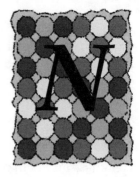

Narcotics

A narcotic is defined in the dictionary as any drug that dulls the senses, induces sleep, and with prolonged use becomes addictive. This is an antiquated definition that fails to mention the primary reason for using narcotics: *to relieve pain*. A preferable term is *opiate* (any natural or synthetic drug similar to opium in its pain-relieving qualities). In hospice and the care of terminal illness, we have very little—if any—concern about addiction.

> Remember: *Addicts use drugs to "get high" and avoid reality. Terminally ill patients require drugs to provide relief of pain and discomfort so they may better experience reality and improve the quality of life.*

Give opiates on a regular schedule rather than waiting for the patient to suffer pain. This maintains a constant level of medication in the body and prevents pain—which is a better alternative than waiting for it to occur and then having to wait for it to subside. Side effects such as drowsiness, confusion, and nausea are common and will usually disappear in a few days with continued use of the drug. These aren't allergies, and there's no proof that there are any allergies to natural opiates such as morphine.

Be cautious, however, when using narcotics. Withhold the medication if the patient becomes unconscious or unresponsive or has a respiratory rate below 10 to 12 breaths per minute. Morphine is a valuable drug since it is relatively inexpensive, can be administered by several different techniques, and is also available in sustained-acting forms.

Most physicians don't administer morphine or other opiates frequently and may not be familiar with the varying ways it can be given. Physicians who treat the dying are accustomed to the large doses of narcotics that are often necessary to control pain.

Nausea

There are many causes of this disabling symptom: medications, chemotherapy, malignancy involving the liver, stomach, or other intestinal organs, severe constipation, and urinary obstruction are the major things that create nausea.

Although you should make every effort to discover the cause of nausea and eliminate it, extensive diagnostic testing may be a burden, and it may be more prudent simply to eliminate the most usual causes and, if the nausea doesn't go away, treat the symptom. Oral drugs to treat nausea won't be useful if the patient is vomiting. Rectal, transdermal, intravenous, and inhaled antinauseants such as cannabis (marijuana) may help.

I suggest that if you try one medication and it's not effective, add additional drugs of another type until the patient gets some relief. Nausea may actively require a combination of three or four drugs together to get a response.

Neuritis

Neuritis (also called neuropathy) means pathology that involves a nerve. Usually it's inflammation or something irritating the nerve such as pressure caused by inflammation or an invading tumor. The pain of neuritis is often sharp and runs along the course of the involved nerve. It may travel down the legs or arms or in between the ribs as with herpes zoster (shingles). Neuritis is painful and feels like burning. The pain may get worse when the afflicted part is moved or stretched.

There are many different treatments for neuritis. The first step in treating neuritis should always be discovering the cause. In some cases the cause is apparent, such as a tumor infiltrating into or pressing on a nerve. Many times the cause of neuritis isn't so clear, but you may need to try treatment anyway.

Antidepressant drugs (tricyclics) often help a neuropathy. Besides relieving nerve pain, when they are given at night antidepressants can help a patient sleep and relieve the depression that's so common with unrelenting pain.

You might have to resort to nerve blocks or even cutting the affected nerve. Virus infections of nerves such as herpes can strike the eyes, lips, genitals, and anus. Even after the lesions—which first appear as small blisters—are gone, there may be an aching sensation (neuralgia) that persists for a long time.

Nurses

The concept of hospice is probably one of the most holistic approaches to the patient and family. Not only is the family a major part of it, but hospice is oriented toward the "global" needs of the human being who is at the end of life.

Caring and curing are not separated, as they can be in high-technology medicine, where the physician usually cures and the nurse cares. In hospice, the nurse's role is elevated to a major team member in the patient's management. Nurses are the backbone of home hospice care. They make home visits, provide a timely assessment of what's required for proper care, and enable the other members of the hospice team to contribute to the support of the terminally ill.

Nutrition

Nutrition is vital in patients recovering from illness and expected to regain their health. Providing food, liquids, vitamin supplements, and increased calories is necessary for the patient's recovery.

But in terminal illness, patients aren't usually expected to recover, and the same regimen of vitamins and food is wasteful and ineffective. Many patients will lose their appetite and drop weight. Don't force-feed a patient or prescribe foods the patient finds unpalatable. Caregivers sometimes insist that the patient eat, hoping that doing so will restore the patient's health. The only thing that's really getting fed here is the caregiver's denial.

Remember: *The purpose of food in terminal illness is enjoyment, not nutrition.*

Offer food, of course, and provide any food or drink that the patient likes no matter what time it is. But don't *force* food. As long as the patient can swallow, allow any food (ice cream, candy bars, exotic or ethnic foods) without restriction. If the patient can't swallow, he or she may be able to chew and spit out food just to enjoy the taste. Usually the terminally ill patient's sense of taste will diminish. At that point most patients will reject food.

I know it's hard to watch a loved one wither and refuse food or fluid. Lack of appetite is part of the natural winding-down of the body at the end of life. The discomfort that comes with involuntary starvation or food deprivation *does not* accompany this natural process. Allow the patient to decide whether or not he or she wishes to eat and *respect their wishes*. It'll be a tough thing to do, but it's the right thing to do.

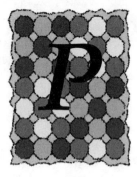

Pain

There are different kinds of pain. Physical pain is a warning that something is wrong with the body. Although we'd like to withdraw—and avoid—pain, it forces us to pay attention to the area that hurts. This makes a lot of sense, since the part that hurts is likely to be the source of the problem, and most of the time we can fix it and make the pain go away.

When the pain is caused by an abscessed tooth, we have the tooth removed or get the abscess drained. This gets rid of the pressure and irritation of the nerve endings and makes the pain diminish. So the first thing we need to do is find out what's causing the hurting. If it's something you can't eliminate (such as invasive cancer), then you must still treat the problem, that is, the pain itself. This is called palliative treatment. It deals with the symptom and not the cause.

Treating the physical pain of terminal illness requires a few steps. First, use enough medication and use it around the clock to suppress the pain enough so that the patient can function. The next thing is to forget all the old myths about morphine and narcotics addiction, and about how pain builds character. These myths are rubbish.

Pain is a destroyer, and only when pain is relieved—whatever its cause—can we address the other painful things associated with the ending of life. Only when physical pain is gone can we deal with the spiritual pain, emotional pain, social pain, and financial pain that comes with dying. These kinds of pain must be relieved to allow the necessary closure of the dying process. Perhaps a more positive way to look at this problem is to say that when physical pain is relieved, there is opportunity for emotional and spiritual growth at the end of life. Physical pain stands in the way of sorting out these other, important problems.

Dying is not "an event"; it is a gradual unfolding of very complicated and intertwined process. It'll take the best efforts of everyone involved for it to proceed to a peaceful end. Severe physical pain doesn't have a place in this process.

These more complex pains can't always be comfortably resolved, and there may be no specific drugs to relieve them (except those that relieve anxiety and depression).

When you're talking to the patient about pain, you need to discover the location and severity—just how bad is it? Mild pain usually needs only mild medicine for relief. A slight headache usually responds to aspirin or Tylenol. (By the way, when I talk about medicine, I'm going to use the trade names, since that's what most people know.)

For practical purposes, divide pain into mild, moderate, and severe or level I, II, and III.

Class I pain can be treated with many drugs. Advil (ibuprofen), aspirin, Tylenol, Darvon, Darvocet, and the like usually provide relief.

Class II pain will need stronger drugs that have an opiate as one of the ingredients. Tylenol with codeine, Percodan, Percocet, and Vicodin are the common examples. These drugs are usually a combination of several drugs and may require a special prescription because of the federal law regulating controlled substances.

Class III pain almost always requires a strong narcotic such as morphine or Dilaudid.

Physicians who don't have a lot of experience with pain management—particularly helping to relieve pain in dying patients—tend to underprescribe or ration strong pain medicine. This is usually because of unwarranted fears of addiction, substance abuse, potential for overdose or fear of scrutiny by the Drug Enforcement Administration (DEA). Doctors inexperienced with pain management also prescribe lower than effective doses simply because of their lack of experience with the pain suffered by the dying patient.

There are situations where the doctor may begin early using small amounts of a potent drug to help mild pain. This is probably a wise move, since the patient may need to have the dosage slowly ramped up as pain worsens. An increase in pain doesn't always mean that the disease is getting worse or that the end is near. There is no upper limit to the dose of drugs such as morphine—use the dose that works for as long as it's needed.

Most patients will get relief from medication given by mouth—medication by injection is painful, irritating, and not necessarily more effective.

Once there is no physical pain, the patient can focus on the resolution of (or accommodation with) the other matters. The patient will need to complete and resolve personal relationships, reconnect with spiritual concerns, and finally to adjust to the idea—and the powerful reality—of life's end.

Dying is both a complex and yet paradoxically simple process. Understanding the diverse nature of human beings, and dealing with all the facets of the dying person's life, makes the end of life the final stage of growth.

Remember: *Pain is subjective—if a patient says he hurts, believe it.*

Terminally ill patients have the right to expect good pain control. Patients should not have to "earn" their morphine.

Suffering in the presence of effective pain-relieving medicine is inexcusable.

Palliation

When we can't cure, we treat the symptoms of the disease. In hospice terms *palliation* means treating the pain, relieving the symptoms, and removing—to the best of our ability to do so—the patient's distress over these things. Treating a patient to improve abnormal lab results, or reduce the size of a tumor on an X-ray may be encouraging to the physician, but it's worth little to the patient who is suffering.

Palliation means "to cloak or cover" and must deal with what the *patient* needs "cloaked or covered." The patient needs relief from pain and symptoms that are uncomfortable or disabling. The patient needs us to make it possible to use fully the end of life.

Pets

Pets seem to know when something is amiss. They seek comfort and reassurance from those who are sick, in the process giving back to the patient more than they take. When I'm sick in bed, my cats and dogs seem to hang around the me more and camp out in the bedroom. In my home visits I frequently encounter pets under, on, and in the bed with the dying person.

There are two times in our lives when touch is crucially important: when we are infants and when we are at the end of life. The closeness of a pet and the intimacy that the contact provides is valuable to terminally ill patients.

Physical Signs of Dying

We can't predict *exactly* when death will occur. There are some signs you can use to determine if the end of life is near. The patient may withdraw, be inattentive, and express no interest or response to stimuli. The patient may sleep more and even fall abruptly asleep. Many patients refuse food and fluids in the weeks or days before death. If the patient's body is still responsive to irritants, body temperature may elevate from infections or due to cancer. Closer to death, the patient's body temperature might not be as reactive, and may even drop.

Blood pressure falls and urinary output decreases before death. The patient's pulse may slow, but most of the time, it becomes rapid, thready, and sometimes irregular. The dying person's skin may become clammy, and it can turn waxy-looking and bluish. The nailbeds may develop a dusky color (a sign of low blood pressure, slow circulation, and less oxygenation in the lungs).

If the patient's breathing is impaired, he or she may appear flushed from the accumulation of carbon dioxide in the lungs. Few of these signs require treatment.

Deep and rapid breathing alternating with times of no breathing (Cheyne-Stokes respiration) is common. Observers may find this worrisome—particularly when breathing stops. The so-called "death rattle" that we see in the hours before the end isn't

71

always present. You can reduce it by administering medications such as atropine, avoiding excess hydration, and not forcing fluids on the patient. Sometimes it's hard to remove the secretions that gurgle in the patient's airway, since they're usually beyond the reach of most suction devices. The "rattle" is probably more distressing and annoying to the caregivers than to the patient.

Days to hours before the end, patients may become less responsive and slip into a coma from which they cannot be roused. Moaning during this time doesn't always mean that the patient is in pain. Also at this point you can reduce the amount of pain medication, and perhaps give it by another route (under the tongue or rectally).

Patients may become agitated and restless, hallucinate, change their breathing patterns, and may lie with eyes open while not appearing to see. As the end approaches, the skin can become mottled or blotchy.

Reassurance, touching, talking, and comforting should be extremely helpful (to both caregivers and the patient) during these final moments.

Placebo

A placebo is an inactive substance or "harmless" treatment of no therapeutic value except to satisfy a patient's need for treatment. Whenever we take a medicine that we hope will work, there's at least a 30 percent chance that it will help—that's called the "placebo effect." Sometimes, instead of giving a specific medicine to relieve a symptom, a doctor will prescribe a placebo. Unfortunately, placebos are usually prescribed for patients we don't like and want to prove wrong.

There is no place for placebos in hospice care.

Prediction

We may know that a person is going to die but not be able to predict when. The fact that we know something about the natural history of a disease, or type of tumor, can make our predictions a bit better. The course of any disease can be slowed by therapy.

Other times treatment can aggravate the illness or produce complications that themselves can be life-threatening. This may accelerate the progression toward death. When illness doesn't respond to treatment we're better able to predict life expectancy. Sometimes we can anticipate the end of life in months, sometimes in weeks, and when the changes are rapid, sometimes in days and hours.

Although we're looking at physical death, remember that the timing of the process is affected by social, emotional, and spiritual dying. These emotions and attitudes can accelerate—or inhibit—dying. Sometimes a patient will fight death until after a particular event such as a graduation, a wedding, or the birth of a grandchild.

One of the most frequent questions families ask me during home visits is: "How long do you think it will be?" Usually they hold the question until I'm at the door or on the front porch. Sometimes I can make a rough guess, but usually I'm not accurate unless the patient is in the final days or hours. Hospice nurses are usually better at predictions. I'm not sure why, but perhaps over the course of their careers, the constant honing of the "intuitions" we all have helps them make more accurate predictions of the time of death.

I think most people asking the question do want to know the answer, but unspoken is the need they have of reassurance that they're doing things correctly. They want to know that they'll be able to handle all the unpredictable events as they will unfold. They need to prepare themselves. The family members want to know that they will be able to control the patient's pain and make it through a frightening and uncertain time.

When I hear the question I stop and take a moment to try to relieve their fears and anxiety. Most families do exceedingly well and pull through the process much better than they expected they would. Sometimes caregivers secretly crave that the entire matter would "just end" and then feel guilty about that. Many ambivalent feelings arise during this difficult time.

Don't reprimand yourself if you have such thoughts. The swirling and complex web of emotions most people feel as a loved one dies are perfectly normal. Punishing yourself for being human is a waste of your time and energy. Expend your energy, instead, on making the patient's last days a meaningful experience for you and your loved one.

Pronouncement

The law varies in different parts of the United States as to who may legally declare or "pronounce" death. When a person dies at home, the police are concerned if the death was natural or not. When the authorities and mortuary know in advance that the person was a hospice patient with an attending physician who has recently visited, there's rarely a problem. The physician can sign the death certificate and the legal part of the matter will be closed.

In the state of California, any competent adult may pronounce death. It's usually unnecessary to call the paramedics or the police or to expect a physician or nurse to be in attendance. It's a waste of the professionals' time to be present. Sometimes the physician or nurse might want to be there (if the family needs support). Generally, the lack of vital signs is obvious, and the family can use this time to privately bring things to a close.

Check with the local authorities to be sure you've met all legal requirements and regulations in this respect.

Psychotherapy

It's safe to say most of us at birth didn't get a book of instructions that would see us through life's ordeals. While the experiences of other people might help us, our own life provides the best lessons—if we pay attention.

Death is a unique experience, and one that can peg the stress meter. There's no rule that says we need suffer the stress of experiencing the death of a loved one without outside help. There is help available, and you should look for it, whether the event at hand is your own inevitable death or that of a loved one. You don't have to justify your need for counseling or outside help. If you need it, if the situation is overwhelming you, act on your instincts. Ask for help.

It doesn't show any weakness to ask for help—in fact, it takes a courageous person to open up and work with the feelings that the impending death of a loved one evokes. Anger, depression, a sense of "unrealness," and other feelings can confuse *anyone*.

When you lose someone close to you, feelings from early childhood that have been buried for years can reemerge with surprising power. Trying to hide these feelings is a waste of energy and the loss of an opportunity to grow and strengthen from the crisis of death. Counseling can make confusing things clear and frightening things easier to handle. Don't try to "go it alone"; that decision is almost always more painful than asking for professional or spiritual assistance.

Psychotherapy, talking to a psychologist, and counseling from a skilled social worker can be beneficial.

Remember: *We are only as sick as our secrets.*

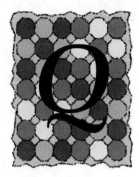

Quality of Life

"Quality of life" is the sum of things that make life valuable and worth living. We use the term a lot in hospice medicine, but it's not easy to define, because it's subjective. What one person defines as valuable and worth every moment may be meaningless to another. Quality of life can't be defined by an observer. It's deeply personal.

There's an old saying that a physician's definition of an alcoholic is somebody who drinks more than the physician. This is a variable yardstick, and it uses the observer as the standard against which everybody else gets compared. It's not a concrete way to define something.

Some people are satisfied with very simple activities, and others feel life is worthless unless they are constantly working and involved in various complicated tasks. Resist the urge to look at a patient and think, *I wouldn't want to live like that.* Guard against the arrogant imposition of your own standards on others. Understand that when a patient expresses the feeling that life isn't worth living, it's not your job to change the patient's mind by denying their feelings.

In the same way that we cannot expect others to die our death for us, neither can we expect them to live our life for us.

Questions

There are always more questions related to dying than there are answers. Patients may wonder why this is happening to them. They may even feel guilty for not having paid attention to early warning signs or having followed through with therapies recommended by their physician.

Caregivers commonly ask some other questions:

Why did this have to happen? Did we do something wrong? Who is at fault? Could this have been avoided? Are we doing things right? Could we have managed things better? What if we make a mistake?

Many of these questions have no clear answer. They are really a way of trying to grasp the enormity of the situation. Death seems so unfair that frequently we look for something or somebody to blame. What these questions are really asking for is reassurance and understanding. There are no stupid or unimportant questions.

Beware of those who appear to know all the answers and have glib responses—they have probably not thought the issue through clearly. A quick and clever response often indicates that the person giving the answer simply wants to avoid the question and is uncomfortable with it.

Feel free to ask health professionals questions. You have a right to an honest answer, and you should feel comfortable seeking a second opinion.

Patients and family are often angry about the things happening to their loved one and may pose their questions in an angry (or even accusatory) fashion.

As a health professional, I try to remember that all questions deserve a sympathetic answer, and I attempt to have a solid understanding of the pain that hovers beneath the surface and often drives anger. I try not to take angry questions personally. I don't always succeed. Sometimes I get defensive when I'm challenged. Take that golden moment between what you feel and your response to remember to answer from a position of love and empathy. This is easier said than done.

Remember: *An empathetic response lessens emotional pain just as opiates lessen physical pain.*

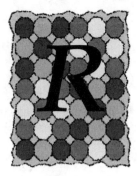

Radiation

The use of radiation and radioactive material to treat cancer is an accepted part of medical practice. Radiation can cure some tumors, reduce the size of others, and diminish their activity. It is also relieves symptoms such as bone pain.

As with all treatments, there are side effects. There may be swelling of surrounding tissues and local inflammation. Some side effects are immediate, and some occur months after therapy. Therapy usually lasts for a few weeks to reduce the intensity of long-term side effects. It's the *total amount* of radiation (measured in various ways) that determines the treatment level, and it can be administered in intense bursts or gradually over time. Some of the delayed side effects may not occur in the limited lifetime of the hospice patient, so the extended treatment may not be appropriate. It might be better to give larger doses over a shorter time.

Just as with chemotherapy, ask questions about radiotherapy before the treatment has started. Expect clear answers. Examine the benefit-to-risk ratio. The benefits should always outweigh the risks in favor of improved quality of life.

Rashes

A rash is a common name for skin inflammation. Usually the rash causes redness and itching, but it might also appear as hives or blisters such as those we see with herpes (shingles, cold sores). You can avoid or lessen many rashes by keeping the skin dry and meticulously clean. Body areas that are warm and moist, such as under the breasts, under folds of fat, in the armpits, and in the groin are where monilia (thrush, candida) will grow.

Bathing, powdering, and using topical antibiotics and anti-inflammatory medications (steroid creams) should help skin rashes. Medications also cause skin rashes. The culprits are usually drugs that have recently been administered. Make an effort to keep each treatment specific, and avoid "shotgun" techniques. An experienced person should make the diagnosis before you treat the rash. Incorrect medication can worsen the rash and increase the patient's discomfort. (Putting steroid cream or menthol ointment on a fungal infection is a good example of this common mistake.)

Reactions to Medicine

Managing terminal illness requires that you take an inventory of and reevaluate all medications. Medicines that were once important may longer be needed. Look at the drugs being given to the patient and determine which are required and which are not.

Diuretics that increase salt loss and lower blood pressure may deplete the patient's sodium and potassium levels. Oral drugs to treat diabetes can often be discarded in terminally ill patients who've lost weight or don't eat. These drugs can cause the blood sugar level to drop (hypoglycemia).

Older, fragile patients can react badly to "the usual doses" of drugs and may need a smaller dose. Not all reactions to drugs are allergies—but all drugs have potential (and sometimes unpleasant) side effects. Keep an eye out for them before they become severe or cause discomfort to the patient.

When a new symptom begins shortly after administering a new drug, it's probably the drug that caused the reaction. If the medication is needed and the side effect is mild or tolerable, it's probably best to continue using the drug. An essential medication is Dilantin (phenytoin), used to prevent seizures. The seizures prevented by the drug would probably be more damaging to a patient than the side effects the drug produces.

Obviously, the physician, in consultation with the nurse and pharmacist, should make the decisions regarding medication. Some drugs must be tapered down and cannot be stopped abruptly without endangering the patient. My experience says that many people have stockpiled numerous medications in their homes that they should sort out. They should probably throw away most of the stockpile, also. The fewer medications the better.

I still believe the best advice is: *"When in doubt, leave it out."*

Respite

A respite is a pause, a period of rest and separation for the patient and for the caregiver. It lets them both rebuild energy and stamina and gives both a break from stress. Everybody involved in the experience of dying becomes depleted—both physically and emotionally. And this includes the patient.

The caregiver and patient may require time to recuperate and gain perspective. They will then be better able to devote energy to the tasks that need doing at the end of life. Respite is essential. It is *not* a luxury. The East Indian poet Rabindranath Tagore once said,

There are two things which man cannot look at continuously, the sun and death.

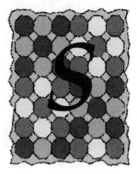

Sadness

I realized that this book would be incomplete without some discussion of sadness. Feeling low in spirit and heavy-hearted is a good way to describe this state without joy. Actually, I can't think of an exact word to describe the feeling, yet when someone says that they are feeling sad, most of us know exactly the feeling. It's as if a dark blanket is draped over us. It's something we just can't shake off, and life just doesn't feel okay when this shroud is clinging to us.

Thirty-five years ago, when I was in medical training, I was assigned a new patient. She was a lovely young woman who came to the clinic for a stress-related muscular problem. Recently, I made a home visit on the same patient. She has widespread cancer of the breast. She's lost weight, she's too weak to talk, her hair is grey, and she is partially paralyzed. She is dying.

I felt incredibly sad as I left her house, waving good-bye through the window as I walked down the stairs. I realized that her dying not only represented the end of her life, it represented the end of a piece of *my* life. I was forced to look at her aging and her end and reflect on mine. It was so long ago when I first met her, yet it seemed to me as if it were yesterday.

I tried to make some sense of it, but for me the best thing to do is to just experience the feelings. This will help to heal the pain.

Sadness is a normal human response to loss. Problems happen when we don't allow ourselves to experience emotions such as sadness. Instead of automatically rejecting powerful and perhaps unpleasant emotions, we should examine them, perhaps embrace them, and just allow them to be.

Sedation

Sedation is a common side effect of many drugs. Antihistamines and antianxiety drugs may produce sedation. Some antidepressants have this effect, and this is the primary effect of hypnotic drugs and sleeping medications. Morphine, intended to relieve pain, may also cause sedation. The fact that pain is now gone (or at a manageable level) may allow the patient to rest and catch up on lost sleep.

While sedatives may make patients less troublesome, they also diminish the experience of living. Sedation may be required to reduce extreme anxiety or agitation. You might also have to accept sedation as an unavoidable side effect from a necessary drug. Maintain a balance between the desired effects and the undesired side effects. Remember this: *Do not sedate and tranquilize patients to relieve the anxiety of the family or caregiver.*

Sleep

As the end of life approaches, patients tend to sleep more. They may even fall asleep during conversations or while being bathed. You may have to interrupt the patient's sleep to keep their care and medicine schedules on time. Patients who wake up at night may be concerned when it's hard for them to fall back asleep. Assure them that even through they're not sleeping, they're getting rest. Also be sure you've done all you can to relieve pain and suppress other symptoms that can interfere with sleep.

Patients may sleep more when you administer a new drug such as morphine. As they become used to the drug, the drowsiness will pass.

Sleep is a comfortable way for life to end.

Smell

Terminal illness may alter the patient's sense of smell. Sometimes the altered smell may disturb the patient. Taste and smell are tied together, so how the patient perceives food can be affected by changes in how things smell. At this writing, there is no effective remedy that can restore the sense of smell (unless it's caused by a nasal or sinus infection that we can treat).

The smell of a dying patient as experienced by those caring for the person may be bothersome, too. Breath odor, vaginal discharge, perspiration, infection in skin creases under the breasts, colostomy drainage, fecal soiling of bedclothes, wound drainage, bedsore breakdown, and urine all cause offensive odors. These smells compound the problems in managing patients. Patients may be deeply embarrassed by body odor. Do whatever you can to keep patients clean and deodorized. They need to be reassured, and they need to be touched.

Remember: *You can always wash your hands.*

Hospice professionals may be able to suggest products and methods useful for reducing and eliminating offensive smells.

Spiritual Pain

Spiritual pain is difficult to define. We immediately think of God, religion, or church. A simple and useful definition for me is that spiritual means "having and expressing spirit." By spirit, I mean the quality of *aliveness*—the essence of life that we express because we are human beings.

I'm aware that this isn't a strict medical definition, nor is it one with which everyone will agree. It's evident that when people begin to slip away from life, many lose their spirit—they become dispirited and something seems to leave them. Becoming dispirited is painful.

Sometimes relieving spiritual pain requires that we help the patient rekindle the ability to appreciate each moment of life. Hospice is dedicated to improving the *quality of life*. Because of this, addressing spiritual pain is important. Some people believe that spiritual pain is caused by loss of contact with God or connections to a particular religious group. Other people want nothing to do with organized religion. This doesn't mean that they do not suffer spiritual pain.

Some people enjoy recalling joyful events in their life, and through this, they relive the meaningful experiences they've had.

Most of us would like to think we've done good things, that we were special in some way, or *we made a difference* because of our presence. Regret at the end of life is often for the things that we have not done rather than the things we have done.

Review the patient's lives with them, and emphasize the positive milestones and pleasant memories. Taking the time to do this can help relieve pain of the spirit. Seek out and talk to a minister, priest, rabbi, or shaman. Their area of expertise is in healing spiritual pain and offering an opportunity for spiritual growth.

Stiffness

Patients who are bed-bound and inactive suffer from stiff joints. This can be either in the arms and legs or in the spine. The stiffness can be worse in patients who have been paralyzed by a stroke or brain tumor. Stiffness is also present in patients who have a preexisting neurological disease such as Parkinson's disease. Joint stiffness tends to worsen with inactivity and only constant attention will keep the joints mobile.

Regular gentle exercise, passively moving the arms and legs through their range of motion, stretching, and applying heat may stop progressive tightening and contractions. Consult with a physical therapist if you're not sure how to do these things.

Suffering

Pain is caused by stimulation of receptor nerve endings in the body that transmit impulses to the brain. Pain notifies the brain that something is wrong. When we notice an uncomfortable sensation, we try to withdraw from it. When we can't withdraw or remove the source of pain, we try to alleviate it with medications. We commonly use aspirin, acetaminophen, codeine, morphine, and so on to help pain.

Suffering is more than just a response to pain—it's the enduring, the tolerating, or the bearing of pain. Suffering means all the unpleasant stuff that comes with pain, such as fear, anxiety, and fatigue.

I think of pain as a chain. The first link is pain itself, the actual *feeling* of hurt. The next link is *suffering* the pain, if it can't be made to go away. The final link is *anguish*—when the pain becomes more than the person can bear. Anguish can deeply threaten the quality of the person's life. It's much more than an annoyance; it is when pain becomes the only thing the person can be concerned with.

Enduring pain and experiencing suffering and anguish are unnecessary. They also waste valuable time—something in short supply at the end of life. We should do anything we can to control pain and maximize the patient's ability to experience fully the remainder of life.

Remember: *Pain does **not** build character. Suffering is **not** a saintly virtue.*

Surgery

Consider the aim of any surgery before it is performed. Many surgical procedures can increase comfort and help the patient live longer and enjoy a better quality of life. Surgery to relieve a bowel obstruction, repair a hip fracture, plastic repair of large bedsores—all these can improve the patient's life when they're used properly.

If you can make the patient comfortable with less invasive and traumatic procedures, don't choose surgery. Decisions about surgery are difficult, and it's not always possible to know in advance if the choice to perform—or not perform—was correct. Nobody can predict all the possible outcomes of surgery. Nor can anybody claim to know every consequence of not performing the procedure. None of us has access to a crystal ball.

These complex decisions should be made with the cooperation and full participation of other medical professionals, the patient's family, and the patient. The patient should be informed of all the options and all the possible (and likely) results. Even if the surgery makes the patient's condition more grave—or if the patient dies after the procedure or after the decision to not perform surgery—you should be able to say that you made the best choice under the circumstances.

Don't allow an unfortunate and unwelcome outcome to cause you to blame yourself (or anyone else) for what happened. Do not feel guilty if your best efforts fail.

Swelling

Swelling, usually caused by fluid accumulating in the tissues beneath the skin, can occur anywhere in the body. Swelling may worsen if the patient takes in salt or salty foods. Kidney failure can cause swelling, also, because malfunctioning kidneys won't be able to excrete salts.

Sometimes diuretics can reduce swelling, or edema. Use diuretics cautiously, since they can reduce blood volume and blood pressure, as well as deplete the body of electrolytes such as potassium. Lowered potassium levels may make the patient weak, or worsen existing weakness.

The physician must first determine what's causing the swelling. There may be no effective treatment for swelling if it's caused by an obstruction of venous blood flow, a lymphatic obstruction, or by a tumor.

Many patients suffer from swelling of the feet, ankles, and legs. This is made worse by prolonged sitting with the legs suspended below the patient. You can help this type of swelling by having the patient lie in bed with his or her legs elevated above body level.

Talking

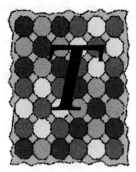

While speaking at a meeting of hospice professionals in Georgia in late 1991, I told a story I'd like to repeat here. I visited a woman who has breast cancer. She had undergone all the treatment available for her cancer. She was at home, and would likely die at home. I asked her to talk with me about her experiences since she had gotten the diagnosis of terminal cancer.

She said, "I've always been a pretty straightforward person, and I want to know exactly what's wrong with me. I'd rather know than not know, and I think that most people would want it that way." I asked her if people treated her differently after they found out that she was dying, and in what way were they different. She told me, "Oh, I can tell. There's a shift—they avoid talking about my illness, and they never ask me about the prognosis. I know it's upsetting for some people, I can understand that. But I would think that they'd talk about the things that are important to me. They treat me differently, they act as if I'll break. They 'fragilize' me. It makes me wonder, just how deep our friendship goes when they keep avoiding the subject…

"I know," she continued, "that no one is completely at ease with my dying. In fact, I think that they would be disrespectful if they were completely at ease—like they took this special event for granted."

We talked about all the things that friends and loved ones could say. She told me that one of the sad memories that still lingers is that she never had a chance to say good-bye to her husband before he died. Before I left, I told her that I hoped when I said good-bye at the end of the visit, she wouldn't mistake my meaning. We laughed about this.

I felt her openness and honesty would make a difference in the lives of people who read what she had to say. So the question remains, in the minds of many people: *How do you talk to the dying*? The answer is easy: *the same way you talk with the living*.

Take the time to affirm and validate your friendship. Share memorable experiences from the past. Talk about the meaning of a person's life—the little things and the big things that make us feel special. Say things like, "I love you." These are the things we assume the other person knows—but often we leave them unsaid. Express your feelings freely. Clean the slate of things you have always felt needed finishing. Be there for this special person, just the fact that you are there means something.

Say good-bye. Tell them you are sorry they are dying. Tell the dying person you will miss them, that you are sad, that you will be lonely without them. Mention the good times you have had with this individual. If you can't manage any of these, say simply, "I don't know what to say." It's a myth that we should always be nice and never say unpleasant things to a dying person. There are times when we can share our hurts, losses, missed opportunities, and frustrations about the past without "dumping." This can sometimes provide for some healing.

Death is a special once-in-a-lifetime experience, and it's not something that most of us look forward to. Most people have fears about death and don't want to talk about it. That's why we avoid the "D" word and talk about *life* insurance rather than what it really is, *death* insurance. Woody Allen once said, "I'm not afraid of death, I just don't want to be there when it happens."

And, sometimes, it's not death itself that brings fear, it's the process of getting there. Fear hides in the shadows created by keeping something a secret. Talk openly with the dying person and bring these things into the light where they can be banished.

Remember: *You have nothing to lose but fear itself.*

Teeth, Gums, and Dentures

As patients lose weight and become debilitated, their gums may shrink and recede. Teeth may loosen, and dentures might fail to fit comfortably. Keeping up mouth care is important, not just for hygiene, but also because it affects whether or not the patient can eat. They can't eat, enjoy the taste of food, and maintain their appearance if their oral care isn't adequate.

Remember: *Modesty and vanity aren't lost with the advent of terminal illness.*

Telling the Truth

Sometimes friends and family may believe that a terminally ill patient shouldn't be told the truth, and should be spared the bad news about their illness. People fear that the patient won't be able to stand hearing the facts, and that irreversible depression will follow. Many people are afraid that the knowing that an illness is terminal will hasten death.

People who believe these things have forgotten something very simple: humans have a built-in "buffer" called "denial." People will not hear what they cannot accept. More accurately, they hear the information, but the mind doesn't register the unacceptable data. Sometimes the unwanted information never gets in, and denial rules the patient's life until the end.

Truth *will* set us free—after we've gotten over the upset and anger it can bring with it. This is the normal way we deal with things we don't want to hear. To withhold the truth from a patient might be for our protection—and not in the patient's best interest. Lying is not telling the truth, and withholding information is also not telling the truth—it's just a passive way to lie. It robs patients of choice and prevents them from choosing how they wish to spend the rest of their life.

Remember: *It is their life and their choice, not ours.*

There are situations where patients are demented or too gravely ill to make any meaningful choice. In these cases, absolute honesty and providing truthful information isn't valuable. I think most patients know what's going on, even if it's at a deep unconscious level.

Often there's a "conspiracy of silence" between the patient and family, with everyone pretending to ignore the way things are (for various reasons). It takes a lot of energy to keep secrets, and you would do better to use that energy elsewhere. Hospice professionals shouldn't lie—although we can refrain from offering the truth unless asked about it. Hospice professionals should answer any questions about diagnosis, prognosis, and any other issues related to the patient's care. We are obligated to be honest. Tell the truth as gently as possible. Ask people how much information they want and tell them what they want to know.

These are simple rules, but following them is the best way to maintain integrity and credibility.

Terminal Illness

We use the words "terminal illness" a lot in this book. Because of this, an explanation of what they mean follows. An illness or disease that will bring an end to life is a terminal illness. When we say "terminal illness," we are referring to a medical problem that—if untreated and allowed to follow its usual course—will end in the patient's death within six months.

The problem with this is that a patient may have lung cancer that's incurable, but its growth will slow down if the patient receives chemotherapy and radiation treatment. It's still a "terminal" illness, but there's a good chance that the patient may live five more productive and enjoyable years rather than six months if he or she is treated. In any case, the patient may live much longer than six months.

In this book, what I mean by terminal illness is a disease where there is no further curative treatment. The type of treatment the patient requires is palliative care (treatment of pain and symptoms), and life expectancy is six months or less. Obviously, nobody can predict the time of death exactly. What we're talking about is an estimate that the physician will need to examine and perhaps revise. There are physicians who have said, "I can't tell if the patient has six months or less to live—I'm not God!" That's an obvious fact, of course, nobody but God is God.

So let's rephrase the question you might want to ask your physician: *Doctor, given your knowledge of the natural history of this particular disease, and with our experience and knowledge of this patient, do you have a rough estimate of how long this patient has to live?*

It seems reasonable to me to expect that a physician would sit down with you and help create a prediction of what the future holds for the terminally ill patient.

Thrush

Thrush is another name for monilial infection or candidiasis. It refers to white patches that appear in the mouth and throat of a person infected with this fungus. Monilia may grow in many parts of the body. It's most common in the mouth, pharynx, and esophagus of patients with AIDS. It can occur in the pubic area, the vagina, and in most any place where the skin is warm and moist. White splotches aren't always apparent in the mouth; sometimes there's only a redness (particularly in the corners of the mouth).

Effective treatments include antifungal creams, gargles, and troches. Monilia affects chronically ill patients who've been on antibiotic therapy. Occasionally, monilia can become a systemic illness (it goes into the body). It requires intravenous therapy if that happens. Whether or not you should pursue aggressive treatment of systemic monilia will depend on the general condition of the patient. Weigh the risks of treatment against the potential benefits.

Toilet

Many cultures (including our own) are preoccupied with regular and normal bowel movements. Bowel function changes during life, and certainly isn't "normal" when the patient isn't eating. The volume and frequency of stool will decline in rough synchronization with how much the patient eats. Altered bowel function and difficulty having a bowel movement may worry some patients. Bowel function is slowed or impaired by many drugs, making fecal impaction common in the terminally ill. Establish a bowel program early in hospice care.

When it's possible, provide the patient with a way of handling this matter privately. Also remember it's impossible to change a lifetime of bowel habits without some physical and emotional discomfort. It's an embarrassing subject for many patients, so handle it delicately.

Touching

Touching is important throughout life. When we are used to being touched and it stops, we notice that. Touching, petting, and physical contact is a means of expressing affection, acceptance, and bonding, and it shows a concern for the welfare of the person being touched. It helps reduce the feeling of loneliness and isolation that is common in the dying. Spouses of terminally ill patients may feel awkward and avoid closeness, perhaps afraid they might injure their loved one, who has become frail. Encourage close intimate contact, bathing, feeding, massaging, sleeping in the same bed—and even sex—if it's possible. Any fear of worsening the illness and hastening death is probably unfounded.

Touching a loved one allays their fear—and it provides us with special memories of our companions and friends after they are gone.

Trade-offs in Treatment

It might seem cold and clinical to say that we all have to die of something. But this is true. If we treat sepsis caused by a sudden urinary tract infection in a dying patient, what next? Something will eventually kill *every* patient. As hospice professionals, we're committed to making the road a bit easier—not longer or shorter because of therapeutic detours. A patient dying of hypercalcemia (high body calcium) from a malignancy may not suffer. In fact, patients with this problem become drowsy and are quite comfortable at the end. If we choose to treat this with intravenous saline, the patient may awaken to further pain and severe pulmonary congestion caused by the overabundance of fluids in the body.

In hospice we're not therapeutic nihilists, nor do we advocate squeezing the last bit of life out of the dying. If treating a condition will allow further life with quality—and it's the patient's choice to do so—then we should perform the treatment. If we're treating a condition and the product of our work will be a more uncomfortable death or further pain for the dying person, then we're not doing our best work.

I always find it difficult to be sure if I've made the best choice in deciding whether or not to perform a treatment. When you've considered the alternatives, consulted with experienced professionals, and shared the responsibility for each decision with others, and respected the wishes of the patient, you've done all that you can do.

Tubes

The most common kinds of tubes are feeding and drainage tubes. Tubes are used to drain secretions from the stomach, intestine, or urinary bladder. Tubes can be used to bypass an obstruction and drain the liver and gallbladder. You may have to drain abscesses using tubes, and sometimes you'll implant tubes to recirculate body fluids. The Denver shunt is one of these—it is used to relieve the accumulation of abdominal fluid.

We use tubes for feeding and to provide fluids. They can be intravenous or subcutaneous infusion lines, or they might be nasogastric or gastrostomy (directly into the stomach) feeding tubes.

Feeding and hydration tubes are useful when the patient might recover—or if they might increase the patient's life span *and* the quality of the remaining days. If the only function of the tube is to prolong the dying process (and keep us from appearing negligent), don't use it.

Although outsiders may think that removing or not implementing a feeding (or other tube) is improper, we know better. Of course, you should consider all the legal and ethical issues prior to discontinuing this form of life support. You can avoid this touchy issue only if you clearly examine the reason for using feeding and other tubes before they've been implemented.

Tumors

A tumor is a growth. It usually grows in soft tissue and serves no function. Tumors are also called *neoplasms*, *masses*, or *lesions*. Tumors may be benign (they aren't spreading) or malignant (which means cancerous and actively spreading). Malignancies vary with the type of tumor. They may begin in one form of tissue, invade an adjoining tissue, and spread, called *metastasizing*. They do this through the bloodstream or lymph channels.

Tumors occur in all areas of the body, and you can sometimes feel them under the skin. Some tumors may erupt through the skin, and can be either painless or painful, depending on how much (if any) pressure they exert on sensitive tissues. They can't be contracted by touching. In most cases, a biopsy is necessary to establish the characteristics of the tumor. The results of the biopsy will help guide any decisions on the most effective therapy.

Turning the Patient

Bed-bound patients, particularly those who are poorly nourished or underweight, will develop bedsores (decubiti) if they aren't turned regularly. Turning the patient frequently and using air mattresses may help prevent bedsores, but there's no guarantee bedsores won't occur despite the best care.

Some patients find a comfortable position and refuse to move. Your efforts may fail if the patient picks a comfortable posture in bed and won't move from it. The patient needs to turn to reduce the chance of bedsores developing.

In skilled nursing facilities, health department officials usually attribute weight loss and bedsores to poor care. This might be the case in some places and some individual situations. This isn't necessarily the cause in all cases. You cannot always blame signs of deterioration on poor care.

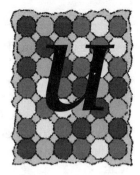

Unfinished Business

Unfinished business is everything that's left incomplete after death. It usually refers to the things left unsaid to the dying person or the things we didn't do. Unfinished business has a nasty by-product: a lingering voice that says, "If only I had…" (finish the sentence however you'd like).

The best time to finish personal business is *before* the patient's death. That prospect can be frightening, for example, saying *I love you*, and expecting to hear *I love you, too*—which may not happen. Completing business doesn't mean making accusations or dumping all your unspoken feelings. It's *sharing* all your feelings with the person who is dying. Even if the person doesn't appear to hear or respond to our words, we need to say them anyway, regardless of the response.

It is *our* business that we need to finish.

Most people believe that we should say only positive and loving things—after all the person is dying. This isn't necessarily so. It's inappropriate, for example, if you don't feel completely loving and positive about the relationship. Many people feel ambivalent. They have mixed feelings. This is a normal reaction.

Saying how we really feel can be healing for us, for the relationship, and for the dying person, who may have an opportunity to explain or to apologize for past mistakes and behaviors. It's a time to make amends.

A young man might say to his father, "Dad, I'm sorry that you're dying, and that I haven't had a chance to get to know you better. I'll miss you. But I won't miss the times you abused me and humiliated me and punished me unfairly."

Saying this doesn't mean that I advocate punishing a dying parent or being cruel. I'm talking about sharing both positive and negative emotions. People should be allowed to die "in character," dying as they have lived. People who have never been kind or loving (for whatever reasons) ought not to be sanctified because they are dying.

If you can't say how you feel to the dying person, it might help you to write a eulogy or a letter that you never mail. Or simply write all your feelings on a piece of paper. That can be very healing.

Remember: *When we complete our unfinished business, we can get on with life.*

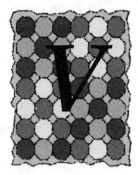

Visitors, Friends, and Family

Sometimes people who haven't been involved in the care of a dying patient try to step in and take over. Usually they do this to get some sense of control, and to ease guilty feelings they may have over their previous lack of interest or participation. As noted earlier, these people may inject themselves into the patient's management, offer advice based on incomplete knowledge or comprehension, and generally become a thorn in everyone's sides. They may recommend new therapies or new consultants, and push their own agenda for straightening things out. Most people who do this mean well and have good intentions.

Other "concerned bystanders" are simply ignorant, self-serving, or frightened. They will cause turmoil and interrupt the path to a smooth closure for the patient and family.

People such as this are difficult to deal with, and even harder to ignore. Remember that advice is cheap, and when you accept such advice, you usually get your money's worth. It's important to consider with care any suggested treatment changes. If a friend suggests a new test or more X-rays, ask this question:

What are we going to do with this new information?

If you're going to embark upon a more aggressive treatment plan, it might not be worth gathering more (and expensive) data just to satisfy curiosity. Well-meaning friends and family may offer suggestions because they feel helpless and need to do something. The point here is that suggestions from others about treatment must really answer the following questions:

1. Is this what the patient wants or would have wanted?
2. If we find another medical problem, will it be worth doing more tests and treatment? Will this really make a difference?

3. Since we know the person is dying, will more tests and treatments improve the quality of life? Or will they take up more "living time" and just prolong dying?

If you have decided that the terminally ill person is to die at home, stick to that decision and use your energy to make this a meaningful and valuable experience for everyone.

The act of letting people come into your home lets them see aspects of you they have not seen before. They see you as part of a family, where you eat and sleep, the books you read, and the things you collect that have special meaning to you. It brings people closer to you, and they get to know you better. They get a more solid sense of the meaning of your life, and a better understanding of the end of your life. You also give visitors a gift by allowing them to share with you, do things for you, and observe your human qualities—things that aren't always seen by friends or business associates.

As the end approaches, visiting times may need to be limited, since "entertaining" guests can be fatiguing for the caregiver as well as the patient who has less energy, a shorter attention span, and needs to sleep more.

Visitors celebrate us. They let us know what we have meant to them, and that we have importance in their lives.

Volunteers

Hospice volunteers are very special people. They offer their services at no charge and willingly donate their time to help others. Many of them have been through their own death and dying experiences and are able to pass on the legacy of caring from which they benefited. Although the motivation of volunteers is to give lovingly without consideration of reward, they're usually well compensated by enriching the lives of those they serve. In many cases, they actually may get more than they give.

Some people are reluctant to share the privacy of their homes with others. While this is understandable, closing out people at the end of life deprives us from the extra attention and joy visitations bring. It keeps other people from really knowing us by caring for us where we live, surrounded by "our stuff." Letting others into our home and our life can be a very rewarding experience for us and for the volunteers.

I remember making a home visit to an elderly gentleman in east Los Angeles. He was sitting in a small backyard near the garage, and a handsome young man was giving him a shave. The young fellow looked like somebody I'd seen on television. As it turned out, he was a volunteer who was also an actor on a daytime soap opera. Both he and his wife were actors who volunteered for hospice. I can think of several glamorous movie stars whom I would choose as volunteers were I in a home hospice program...

Hospice volunteers are exceptions to the rule "you get what you pay for." They are medicine's angels without wings.

Vomiting

Vomiting, or the regurgitation of stomach or intestinal contents, isn't always preceded by nausea. Vomiting refers to the repeated and forceful contraction of the stomach and diaphragm, which then projects the contents of the gut upward, through the esophagus, and out of the mouth.

The ejected matter may consist of digested or undigested food, bile, mucus, or blood. Many causes of vomiting require medical evaluation. Projectile vomiting is sudden, forceful, and without warning. It's sometimes related to and caused by head injury. Whatever the cause, remember that nausea and vomiting are painful, disabling symptoms and require treatment. Often the patient will feel relief only if you administer multiple drugs.

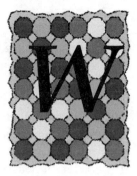

Wheezing

Spasms of the large airways, or narrowing caused by a tumor, swelling, or secretions, can produce high-pitched whistling sounds like those heard in asthmatic patients. The wheezing occurs when the patient exhales, and you can help it by removing secretions with suction, or by administering medications. Sometimes wheezing stems from an allergy or from fluid accumulating in the lungs (as happens with heart failure).

Wheezing is distressing. Some patients wheeze less when they're sitting up. Having them lean forward while breathing through pursed lips may help, too. Wheezing isn't the "death rattle" I mentioned earlier, and should be properly evaluated and treated accordingly.

Wheezing during inhalation could mean there's an obstruction in the upper airway. In this event, consider using suction to remove the secretions that block the flow of air into the patient's lungs.

When to Visit

Friends and family of a dying patient often want to know when they should visit their loved one. Relatives who are visiting from out of town may want to know if they should leave or not. The best advice I can give the caregiver is to tell the relative or friend exactly what the patient's condition is.

Ask the hospice professionals to give you their best assessment on the patient's state. It's usually best for people to arrive too soon to say their good-byes than to arrive too late. This allows them to visit during quality time. Arriving late means there is no chance for a proper closure for the relationship. The important thing is to allow people time for closure before death, even if they must return to their homes before the actual event.

Visitors are responsible for making their own decisions on when to come and how long to stay.

Withdrawal

Patients vary in how much they withdraw at the end of life. Physical withdrawal is shown by decreasing consciousness proceeding to coma. Patients may also withdraw emotionally. I've seen patients turn away from caregivers and refuse to communicate. Some may revert to childlike behavior and hide under the covers. Don't take behavior such as this personally. If the patient is depressed, sometimes antidepressant medication can help. If you use drugs to treat behavioral problems, remember that it's the patient whom you are treating. You ought not to medicate the dying person to lessen your discomfort and your intolerance of their symptoms.

Withholding Food and Fluids

I've addressed this issue in other parts of this book. It's such an important topic that it bears repeating. Not feeding and not providing fluid to a dying patient who doesn't want food or drink (or for whom forced feeding isn't useful) is not the same as withholding food or fluids in patients who are hungry and thirsty. It isn't starvation as we usually define it.

Most dying patients do not experience discomfort if they don't eat or drink. Forcing food and fluids *can* make them uncomfortable.

Part of the dying process is the loss of interest in drinking or taking nourishment. Some of the food supplements designed to provide calories and nourish the sick don't taste good, and the aftertaste they leave isn't the most desirable thing to have lingering in your mouth at the end of life.

When people ask me what food I suggest they offer a dying person, I say, "junk food." That's because I like candy bars and ice cream and cake and pie. So that's my suggestion, if that's what the patient has a taste for, whatever time of day it is when the patient requests something, provide the requested food.

However, if the patient has a problem swallowing, I suggest nothing except good mouth care and lubrication. Forcing food and fluids can make the patient to choke or aspirate and really cause problems.

It's tough to observe a loved one slipping away and not be tempted to "just give them a little something." But that *little something* is more for our benefit than it is for the patient's. Family caregivers and professionals alike have a great deal of difficulty doing nothing and because of this, feeling helpless. Keeping busy keeps us from our feelings, it uses up the time. It's okay to do something—in caring for the dying and there's always something to do—but pushing food and fluids isn't it.

The confusion arises when dehydration and starvation are used as buzzwords to imply that the patient is receiving poor care. This idea causes patients to be inappropriately treated with intravenous fluids, nasogastric tubes, and gastrostomy feedings. The reason behind the treatment isn't to better the patient—it's to relieve guilt or satisfy a misdirected law that won't allow life to come to an end comfortably.

Forced feeding is a waste of resources and serves only to prolong dying. Never forget that you should get competent medical and legal advice before starting (or discontinuing) any treatment.

And remember the most important thing: *Respect the wishes of the dying patient.*

We are talking about, after all, the patient's life—and the patient's death, not our own.

Witness

Few people have been present at the moment when life ceases. This is defined medically when major vital functions stop, and death can be officially pronounced. In most cases, death is the peaceful end of a struggle—a letting go into a gentle rest. It resembles the sleep of a newborn after the rigors of birth.

Friends and family who are present to observe the event may be fearful of the unknown and what their response to it will be. Not many people "freak out" or become emotionally unstable when death happens. Most manage to go through the process with ease, equanimity, and competence.

People don't die as dramatically in the real world as they do in the movies. There's nothing other-worldly about the transition from dying to death. With the best preparation, the moment of death may come as a shock—but it's manageable. We get through it. It seems as if our fears are always worse than reality, and our ability to cope greater than expected.

When my mother died, the nurse was standing at her bedside. She touched my mother's eyelids and said, "It's okay to let go, Helen." And my mother simply became quiet.

For many people, it's important to be present at the exact moment of death. That's just not always possible. I recall a woman who sat at her dying husband's bedside for days on end awaiting his final breath, only to have him die when she took a moment to go to the toilet. She felt cheated, even though she had devoted almost all her time and energy to him at the end. There is the chance, though, that he died when she was gone to protect her from witnessing it. Only he knows for sure.

Although you may not feel this way in the days prior to a loved one's death, helping to ease the path of the dying—and being there at the final moments—can be one of the most meaningful, rewarding things you will experience.

Trust yourself.

The mark
of your ignorance is the depth
of your belief in injustice
and tragedy.
What the caterpillar
calls the end of the world
the master calls a
butterfly.

—"Illusions" by Richard Bach